Okinawa

Diet

A Meal Plan& Some Recipes for You& So Much More

(Delectable Recipes for Okinawa Diet Cookbook for Staying Healthy)

Lucille Hamilton

Published By **Jordan Levy**

Lucille Hamilton

Okinawa Diet: A Meal Plan& Some Recipes for You& So Much More (Delectable Recipes for Okinawa Diet Cookbook for Staying Healthy)

ISBN   978-1-998769-63-6

Legal & Disclaimer

The information contained in this ebook is not designed to replace or take the place of any form of medicine or professional medical advice. The information in this ebook has been provided for educational & entertainment purposes only.

The information contained in this book has been compiled from sources deemed reliable, and it is accurate to the best of the Author's knowledge; however, the Author cannot guarantee its accuracy and validity and cannot be held liable for any errors or omissions. Changes are periodically made to this book. You must consult your doctor or get professional medical advice before using any of the suggested remedies, techniques, or information in this book.

Upon using the information contained in this book, you agree to hold harmless the Author from and against any damages, costs, and expenses, including any legal fees potentially resulting from the application of any of the information provided by this guide. This disclaimer applies to any damages or injury caused by the use and application, whether directly or indirectly, of any advice or information presented, whether for breach of contract, tort, negligence, personal injury, criminal intent, or under any other cause of action.

You agree to accept all risks of using the information presented inside this book. You need to consult a professional medical practitioner in order to ensure you are both able and healthy enough to participate in this program.

Table of contents

Chapter 1: Fundamentals and Origin

The Okinawa Diet has earned a reputation for being a way to eat that increases life expectancy. A lot of fitness enthusiasts see a correlation between this diet and improvements in health. Many people also have adopted the Okinawa weight loss program. What does the Okinawa Diet actually mean? Is it from where did it come?

Origin of Okinawa Diet

"Okinawa Diet," a term that refers to a specific area in Japan's Ryuku Islands (where the largest island is Okinawa), was created. They claim that this island's high life expectancy is due to their unique eating habits.

The Ryuku Islanders' traditional eating habits include 30% yellow and 25% green vegetables, 15% grain, and 30% sugar. Sweet potato is the Okinawans staple food. Apart from that, the Okinawa Diet is very low in fish and high in soy and other legumes. The most popular choice for pork is organic and grass-fed. All edible parts of pigs, including their internal organs, can be eaten. Actually, each Okinawan's annual pork consumption is more than the Japan national average. For instance, in 1979 the average Okinawan consumed 7.7 kilograms of pork, which was 50% more than Japan.

In 1950, Okinawans ate an average of less calories per day, compared to Japanese residents. This means that they ate less grains, rice, wheat, barley, polyunsaturated oils, eggs, poultry, milk, sugars, and grains. They also avoided pickled vegetables and instead ate more legumes as well as sweet potatoes. This led to Okinawans eating almost 70% sweet potatoes.

The Okinawas have followed the traditional Okinawa diet since the 1960's. The traditional eating habits of the Okinawa people have undergone changes over time. Fat intake has been increased. Sometimes, sweet potato was also served with bread and sometimes rice.

Key Principles of The Okinawa Diet

Okinawan diet requires you to pay attention to your hunger, and be aware of your feelings. It requires that you stop eating after you have satisfied your hunger pangs at 80%. It allows you to satisfy your hunger 20 minutes after eating.

The main points of this diet include lowering your calorie intake and decreasing your caloric fat. You can also increase energy by engaging in aerobic exercises and taking in heart-friendly oils regularly.

A Okinawa diet emphasizes eating foods rich in fiber as well as lean meat and plant protein. It also allows you to drink green or black tea as well as water. Further, the Okinawa Diet divides food items into four distinct categories. The number of calories contained in food items determines the grouping.

Featherweight

These foods have 0.8 calories/gram or less. These include citrus fruits like cucumber and spinach. These can all be consumed in large quantities per day.

Lightweight

These food items have 0.8-1.5 calories per grams and should be consumed with moderation. This group includes potatoes, bananas, and potatoes.

The middleweight

The caloric densities of middleweight foods are 1.5 to 3.0 cals per gram. It is therefore recommended that food items belonging to this category, such legumes and lean meat, be limited in their consumption.

Heavyweight

Many fats and oils, including red meat, oil seed, and nuts, are heavyweight foods. They have a caloric density of 3 to 9 calories a gram and should be avoided.

The Okinawa Diet has one main goal: to reduce calories by paying more attention nutritionally dense foods with lower caloric densities. This means that foods belonging to the lightweight and featherweight category must be the mainstay of your meals. This is vital to lower the risk of overeating, which leads to high levels of calories.

Average Okinawa Diet followers consume 500 fewer calories per day than others. Okinawan food selections are healthy and limit your calories. These foods are low in calories and high in nutrients. They also have low levels of glucose.

Chapter 2: Health Benefits

The Okinawa Diet has many great features that can be used to help people lose weight and improve their overall health. Recent studies show that the Okinawan diet has the potential for improving one's physical well-being. We will be discussing the health benefits of the Okinawa Diet and how it works.

The Okinawans are known for their positive eating habits that have had many benefits over the years. You can expect weight loss, healthier bones, better heart health and normal menopause. Let's explore these positive outcomes.

Weight Loss

The Okinawa Diet is proven to be effective in helping individuals lose weight, according to numerous sources. People who followed the Okinawa diet were able lose excess fat by cutting down on their daily calorie intake. Due to the high-nutrient foods, they were less likely to get overweight-related diseases such as diabetes and hypertension.

Lower Chances of Contracting Cancer

The Okinawa Diet reduces the risk of developing hormone dependent cancers. It does this by consuming fewer calories and more good fats, vegetables, fruits, and other foods. One reason is the large use of turmeric within the Okinawa Diet. The herb has been shown to cure and prevent various types of cancer.

Better Heart Health

Green tea has been proven to be beneficial in preventing certain types of cardiovascular disease, according to some research. Sanpin, Okinawan Green Tea, is a different form of green-tea because it contains more antioxidants than regular green tea. It is also unsweetened. These features make Okinawan tea one of most useful heart health preventives. The Okinawa Diet is also known to help keep the blood vessels in good condition and the bad cholesterol levels low. This reduces one's vulnerability to heart disease by 80%. It is particularly evident for those over 80.

In 2007, Okinawans had a lower risk of getting cancer or heart disease than Americans. It was discovered that Okinawans are 80% less likely be to die from heart diseases than Americans. They are also 70% less likely not to die of prostate cancer.

Improved Bone Health

As you may already know, calcium plays a key role in maintaining bone strength. The Okinawa Diet contains many food groups rich in calcium. Okinawa Diet members are more likely to be protected against fractures and broken bones. This is crucial because every person's bone density eventually decreases. The Okinawa Diet can help you combat it.

Normal Menopause

Women who follow the Okinawa Diet as a woman are less likely to have serious health problems, such as heart disease and osteoporosis. They don't need any hormone replacement therapy or other treatments. This is due to the fact that soy, a major Okinawan dietary item, contains phytoestrogens. These substances are natural and non-toxic, helping to reduce the effects of menopause.

Long Life Expectancy

Because of its promise of longer life expectancies the Okinawa Diet has become very popular. Okinawaians hold the record for having the longest life expectancy. Because of their lifestyle, and the amount of physical activity they do, they are well protected from autoimmune and inflammatory diseases.

The Okinawa Diet - Main Features

The Okinawa Diet, in summary, is a healthy and nutritious eating program. It's a low-calorie, high-quality diet that is rich in antioxidants, low amounts of sugar and saturated fat, and abundant vegetables and seafood.

Low Calorie Diet

The Okinawa Diet, like the others, is calorie-restricted. The Okinawa diet has 20% less calories per gram than the Japanese standard of eating. It is normal for people to consume less than one calorie per gram of bodyweight. A typical Okinawan has a Body Mass Index of 20. As long as you don't restrict calories, it can improve your health and slow down the aging process.

High in Antioxidants

The Okinawa Diet contains green, yellow, and orange vegetables, roots and fruits. It is therefore considered to be an antioxidant rich diet. Okinawan food is rich in antioxidants. These vitamins and minerals protect cells from damaging free radicals and inflammation.

Low in Fats and Sugar

The Okinawa Diet is low in fat, but high in Omega-3 fatty acid, an essential nutrient for fighting cardiovascular diseases such stroke. It recommends a lower intake of saturated and sugary fats, as well as 25%

sugar intake and 75% consumption of grains. This is crucial because a lower sugar intake leads to lower blood sugar levels. A low blood sugar level helps prevent pro-inflammatory body states, which in turn can lead to chronic disease.

Seafood and Vegetables are abundant

Vegetables are and seafood are the two best foods for nutrition. These are two of the most basic Okinawan meals. These basic Okinawan food include a high intake of soy, low-carb vegetables such as bitter melon and legumes, and little or no dairy or poultry products. A lot of attention is given to seafood which is rich in essential nutrients like alpha, eicosapentaenoic and docosahexaenoic. All of this helps to prevent heart and colon problems, as well as prostate and colon cancers.

Chapter 3: Recommended Foods

The best way to explain the diets of these people is to give a list. The Okinawa Diet is described in this chapter. It will be obvious that this chapter does not contain all Okinawan cuisines. It simply lists the main and most nutritious Okinawan meals.

Researchers have discovered that the most popular Okinawan functional foods are among the many. Functional foods are those that can offer health benefits, as well as meeting the basic nutritional macronutrients. Functional foods can include foods that contain phytochemicals that help fight diseases.

These are the thirteen most important Okinawan foods:

Sweet Potatoes, Yams

Americans prefer sweet potatoes to yams, and Japanese love sweet potatoes. Sweet potatoes, yams, and other yams contain high levels of vitamins C, B and A. They are also rich sources of fiber, magnesium, iron and potassium.

Sweet potatoes are Okinawa's most staple food. They are eaten as an accompaniment to rice and are eaten daily. This custom is rooted back in the past, when rice was only a luxury item for Japan's wealthy. Before rice was more expensive and sweet potatoes more affordable, It's good to know that sweet potatoes are less expensive and packed with nutrients and vitamins. Sweet potatoes are recommended by those with type 2 diabetes or high cholesterol.

Soy

Okinawans consider soy their main source of plant protein. Soy is rich in phytochemicals, like phytoestrogens, flavonoids and phytoestrogens. These phytochemicals have health-promoting benefits. Most often, soy is consumed in the form miso paste or tofu.

Studies have shown that Okinawan's tofu is less water- and better fat-rich. It is thicker, harder, more intact, flavorful, and more flavorful then regular Japanese tofu. Furthermore, Okinawans tofu is high in isoflavone. It is associated with low breast and prostate cancer rates on the island.

Goya

The Okinawa Diet includes Goya, which is for Japanese people, and bitter melons for Westerners. Due to its bitter flavor, it isn't usually eaten alone, but is instead incorporated into salads, stir-fried dishes and teas.

Goya is known for its ability to burn fat. Although the bitter taste of raw, bitter melon might be a problem, it is a good way to lose fat. Goya's CLA content, which is conjugated linoleic, or CLA, is said to decrease the accumulation and increase the lean mass. Goya is rich in vitamin C and fiber which facilitates digestion. It's also a common medicinal herb in other nations.

Shiitake Mushrooms

Shiitake mushrooms, which are often found in Asian dishes, are a large type of fungi. They are nutritious and very healthy. Shiitakes are similar to other types of mushrooms. However, they have very low calories and high amounts vitamins A, C, D, and B12 as well antioxidants. These mushrooms also contain a large amount of proteins with all eight essential amino acids. These mushrooms have two important health benefits: they can boost the immune system, and regulate cholesterol.

Shiitake mushrooms are recommended in Japan for their anticancer properties. Researchers have shown that Shiitakes improve survival rates in patients suffering from stomach or pancreatic carcinomas.

Seaweeds

Okinawa's people eat three kinds of seaweeds, kombu, mozuku, and katsuobushi. They are often eaten in salads along with vegetables and noodles.

Seaweeds are functional Okinawan foods because they contain high amounts of iron, calcium, magnesium and iron.

Seaweeds can be used as a natural cure for illnesses such arthritis, colds, flus, and even cancer.

The fat-burning properties of mozuku and other seaweeds are also supported by this. Muzuko's high levels of fucoxanthin (a carotenoid which can help get rid of fat) are a boon. It does this by burning fat from the visceral and keeping the internal organs intact.

Konnyaku

Konnyaku is a jelly made from Konjac. It's common in Japan's islands. It has low fat and caloric densities. It's also high in fiber and calcium. These nutrients help improve bone health, as well as aid in digestion. Konnyaku contains 90% water, 10% glucomannan and 10% soluble fiber. This component makes Konnyaku an effective treatment for constipation.

Konnyaku can also be used to clean the stomach.

Luffa/Loofah or Nebera

Luffa, also known as Nebera, is rich with folate and vitamin B that helps in brain development. It takes some time for the maturation process to be complete so it is only possible to grow in locations that have natural vegetation. Luffa is frequently used in miso-based and tempura dishes. It is considered a low-calorie Okinawan veggie because it contains only 16 calories.

Gobo

Gobo can be described as a fibrous root vegetable. Fiber is an essential component of digestion. Gobo is important for maintaining normal bowel movements. It also helps to regulate blood sugar levels, controlling hunger and satiety.

Okinawans often use spices and herbs. These herbs and spices can be used to make your meals more delicious, as well to add nutrients and antioxidants. These five essential Okinawan herbs and spice are: mugwort; hihatsu; fennel and hechima.

Turmeric

Ucchin, also known as turmeric, is a popular Okinawa herb. To avoid dizziness, many people take it in the form of a pill in Japan. There are studies that show turmeric has healing properties. It's used to treat rheumatoid arthritis, combat the growth of more cancer cells, and reduce symptoms of Alzheimer's disease.

Mugwort

Mugwort is also called Fuchiba, Turmeric's spice. Mugwort has many medicinal properties and is used to enhance Okinawan drinks. Mugwort has sedative properties.

Traditional Chinese medicine uses Mugwort for anxiety, depression, restlessness, restlessness, and irritability. Mugwort, which belongs to Artemisia plants, is also known to treat infectious disease like malaria.

Hihatsu

This is a pepper used to cook or prepare food. Hihatsu can be used to treat gout, stomach pains, and other ailments in Okinawa.

Fennel Seeds

Fennel is also known as Ichoba, Okinawa's favorite vegetable and spice. Research has shown that fennel can be beneficial in losing weight, treating heartburn, flatulence, and treating stomach troubles.

Hechima

Hechima is a low calorie vegetable. It is high in folates, vitamin C, protein and carotenoids. These substances are essential in fighting cancer cells as well as reducing the severity chronic disease.

Because Okinawa's food options are abundant, the diet is very simple. They are also readily available in local markets and grocery shops. Knowing which Okinawan food items you should be eating is the first step to understanding the many menu options that you can make with them. Here's a short discussion about three Okinawan main meals. The Okinawa Food Pyramid is used to create the menus. It was developed after two and a-half decades of research.

For breakfast, try the Okinawa Menu

Blueberry pancakes are an Okinawan option for Westerners used to high-calorie breakfasts. This should include soymilk fortified in calcium, free-range, omega-3 fatty acids-rich eggs, fresh blueberries, and whole grain flour. The Okinawan breakfast blueberry pancake is rich in protein, fiber, antioxidants, and other essential nutrients. The best pairing for blueberry pancakes is an Okinawan Green Tea. It's sugar-free, low in calories and packed with disease-fighting flavonoids. Apples can be used as breakfast snacks.

Sample Okinawa Meal Plan for Lunch

On the Okinawa Diet it's best to choose stir-fried tofu, or steam vegetables. You can make steamed vegetables with dark green leafy veggies like asparagus, bok choy, broccoli and bok choy. Baking sweet potatoes or salads can replace rice. Sweet potatoes are more nutritious that white rice due to their high levels of vitamin E and antioxidants. Seaweed and mozuku soup can be served as lunch. It is rich with vitamins and minerals which are believed to improve the immune system.

Sample Okinawa Menu for Dinner

An Okinawan dinner may include a bowl miso soup with cubed Tofu and green veggies. Steamed fish, shrimp and vegetables can also be served with whole grain noodles. It is important to include seafood at least once a week in your diet. Keep in mind that fish with a low caloric density, such salmon, mackerel or sardines, are not recommended.

Do not eat sugary snacks more often than once a week while you follow the diet of the islanders. If you are looking to indulge, set up a "cheat-day," which is a Sunday that allows you to eat as much or as little as you'd like. This will allow you to satisfy your hunger pangs.

You should only eat fresh fruits for your snack between breakfast and lunch. For your afternoon snack, stick of raw or semi-cooked vegetables is a good choice. The sweetened Japanese rice cake mocha is a sweet treat made from pounded rice.

As you can mix and match various Okinawan dishes according to your personal taste preferences, the traditional diet isn't difficult. You must be aware of the caloric content of your dishes and follow the Okinawa Diet guidelines. This diet requires that you eat a lot of Okinawan food, which should be light and featherweight.

Chapter 4: Pros and Cons

The traditional Okinawa Diet can be worth a try, especially if someone is looking for a natural, healthy weight loss method or healthy eating habits. As with any other diet, the Okinawa eating way has its pros and cons. Below you will find both the benefits and disadvantages of the Okinawa Diet. This article will also cover recent trends in this diet, along with the Okinawa Diet's weaknesses.

Positive Things About the Okinawa Diet

The Okinawa Diet's numerous health benefits are highlighted in the second section. These include lowering the risk of obesity-related chronic diseases. These are just a few of the many benefits that the Okinawa Diet provides.

The Okinawa Diet is different than other diets. It encourages eating carbs, but they are low on the glycemicindex and fats, but only from healthy sources. Proteins should be from lean grass-fed meats as well as some plants. Furthermore, Okinawa Diet calorie limits do not ensure optimal nutrition. Okinawan substitutes for the body's daily caloric intake are rich in essential vitamins. Studies have shown that prolonged low-carb and low-fat diets can cause lethargy as well as damage to hormonal functions.

Because it offers a wide range of vegetarian options, it is easily accessible for vegans. While the Okinawa Diet encourages the consumption and consumption of pork, there are other food options that can replace it, like tofu, seaweeds, and other nutrient-dense food products. A daily diet that includes healthy vegetables (10 servings) and fruits (2 servings) is included. This diet is easy to adapt for those who are used to eating a western diet. The Okinawa Diet includes more than 100 recipes that combine Japanese and Western foods. There are a few modifications that can be made to the Okinawa Diet.

Select soy products and soy-made food items. Cubed tofu can be added to stir-fries. You can also replace regular dairy milk by soymilk.

Reduce the consumption of red meat and replace it with high-quality low-calorie seafood. Lentils are another option.

Add mushrooms to your meals and snacks. There are many varieties, such as Shiitake, King trumpet, oyster and King trumpet. You can make mushrooms the star of your meal.

You should eat more vegetables, particularly those that are deep green.

Another positive aspect about the Okinawa Diet? It is sustainable. They are affordable. These foods can be grown right in your own garden if you so choose. You can easily modify this traditional diet.

Most importantly, numerous scientific studies support the Okinawa Diet. Research has been extensive over the years to better understand the Okinawa Diet. These studies focus on the health benefits, the effectiveness of the diet and the best food choices.

This is vital because it's important to know that you shouldn't try anything new with your health and diet. It will provide you with assurance that the diet you are about try is safe, natural, effective.

Negative Points about the Okinawa Diet

There are still some flaws to the Okinawa Diet that must be noted, no matter how wonderful it may seem. One problem with the traditional Okinawa Diet is its lack of emphasis on regular exercise. The Okinawa Diet only covers a diet and does not include any kind of physical activity.

Although regular physical activity is crucial for good health, some foods are not as nutritious as others. Regular physical activity can improve your heart health and muscle and joint health.

Because of all the reports that the diet has the ability to prolong one's life, many people lose sight of the psychosocial factors which may have played an important role in the Okinawans longevity and health. Indigenes are known for their rich culture and active communities. This is most likely why they live longer. Living a happy life is possible by maintaining a healthy social life and striving for a purposeful lifestyle.

Another problem with the Okinawa Diet are the high levels of sodium in certain food items (such as miso, soya sauce, and saltedfish). It is possible to still have a problem with the increased sodium levels of the Okinawa Diet, even though it is high in vegetables and fruits. The Okinawan flavors might not appeal to Westerners and others who are more sensitive to taste. Following a traditional diet can be hard and frustrating at first.

There have been successes and there have been failures with the Okinawa Diet. It is possible to adapt the traditional diet to your specific needs and preferences. While this diet does not provide a comprehensive set of lifestyle factors that can help you live a long and healthy life, it does include some essential lifestyle elements such as exercise and ways to manage stress. The Okinawa Diet is a nutritious eating plan that helps to reduce calories and increase nutrition.

Current Trends Concerning the Okinawa Diet

The Okinawa Diet has been criticized for its shortcomings. Those who follow it are now looking for ways of making up for them. Some diet promoters include exercises into their plans. They understand the importance to lead an active lifestyle in order to lose weight and improve their overall health.

Many Okinawa Diet fans are now starting to form online and offline communities and support groups that allow them to share and discuss their experiences and progress. This is crucial because it allows individuals to have fun, learn from others and exchange information.

Different culinary and nutritional experts collaborated to devise a Westernized Okinawan recipe. This would make Okinawa Diet a more attractive option for Westerners who are more conservative and also reduce the transition time.

What is the Okinawa lifestyle?

The Okinawa Diet is simply the traditional Okinawa food habits. Their unique lifestyle and diet is credited for giving them one of the longest lived lives on the Earth.

Traditional Okinawa food is low in calories, fat and high in carbs. This diet emphasizes vegetables as well as soy products. It also includes small amounts of noodles, rice and pork.

Modernization of food production methods and dietary habits has seen a shift in macronutrient content for the Okinawa Diet. It's still low-calorie, primarily carb-based, but now has more protein as well. Okinawan culture also views food as medicine and uses traditional Chinese medicine. It includes spices and herbs that are known to have health benefits, like turmeric and mugwort.

Okinawan lifestyle encourages regular physical activity and mindful eating.

A mainstream version has been created to encourage weight loss, based on the health benefits of traditional Okinawan food. It encourages the consumption nutrient-dense foods. However, it is heavily influenced and influenced by Western diets.

Although it is well known that the Japanese are the world's longest-lived people, less well known is that there is a Northeast-to-Southwest gradient in longevity, whereby the longest lived of the Japanese are those that inhabit the southernmost islands, known as the Ryukyu Islands (or Okinawa prefecture). Okinawa, which is also the 47th prefecture of Japan has the longest expected life expectancy. This is due in part to their ability not to develop or delay major age-related diseases such as stroke, heart disease and cancer.

Many people believe that Okinawa has a long-lasting longevity advantage due to its healthy lifestyle. This includes the traditional Okinawa diet. Low in calories, but high in nutrition, this diet includes vitamins, minerals, flavonoids, and phytonutrients. However, diet changes after World War II have had a major impact on Okinawans' health. Younger Okinawans are at greater risk of becoming obese and developing other chronic diseases risk factors than the older Japanese. A resurgence in interest among public health professionals regarding the health-enhancing effects of the traditional Okinawan lifestyle and a movement to re-educate young people in this traditional Okinawa style of eating has resulted in a surge in popularity.

Examining the ingredients and cooking style of traditional Okinawan meals can give you insight into the Okinawan lifestyle. This would usually start with Okinawan style miso soup (water. Miso paste. seaweed. tofu. sweet potato. Sweet potato is the primary carbohydrate and not rice, as in Japanese cuisine. Champuru (a stir-fried vegetable dish) is the main course. This includes bitter melon, goya and other vegetables.

A side dish like konbu seaweed (or konnyaku) is also available. This dish is often simmered with a small amount of oil, bonito daashi broth (for flavour), and small amounts fish or boiled meat. Vegetables and tofu are the main ingredients in many cooking styles.

These staples might be served with smaller amounts of fish, pasta, or lean cuts of meats. Nbushi style uses water rich vegetables like Chinese okra, daikon (radish), pumpkin, and miso to season them. Then they simmer in their own juices. Irichi style uses stir-frying as well as simmering. It also includes less watery vegetables, such as burdock and seaweed, dried Daikon, and green papaya. The meal would include freshly brewed sanpin tea (jasmine), and sometimes a small amount local brewed, awamori.

These descriptions of Okinawa's typical meal can help you to see that the traditional Okinawa diet has the following characteristics.

1) High vegetable consumption

2) High consumption of legumes, mainly soy origin

3) Moderate intake of fish products, especially in coastal areas

4) Low consumption meat and meat products

5) Low consumption dairy products

6) Moderate alcohol consumption,

7) Low caloric intake

8) Rich in omega-3 fats,

9) High monounsaturated-to-saturated-fat ratio, and

10) Prioritization of low-GI carbohydrates

Many of these characteristics are also shared with the traditional Okinawan dietary pattern. Not surprisingly, cardioprotective properties have been demonstrated for all three patterns, due in part to the low consumptions of saturated oil. These diets are thought to have other mechanisms such as high intakes of phytochemicals, high antioxidant intake, low GL and lower CVD risk. They also may be contributing to reduced risk for some cancers and other chronic conditions through multiple mechanisms including decreased oxidative stresses. Comparison of the nutritional profiles of the three dietary styles shows that the traditional Okinawan dietary pattern has the lowest amount of fat, especially in terms saturated fat, and the highest level of carbohydrate intake. This is consistent with the high intakes antioxidant-rich and calorie-poor green leafy vegetable and sweet potatoes.

The Okinawan tradition has been rapidly Westernized since World War II. It has also seen a decline in the quality of carbohydrate, with the shift away from sweet potatoes as the most common carbohydrate to higher intakes of white breads, rice, and noodles.

Despite Okinawa's large increase in fat intake during recent decades, Okinawan's current diet is comparable to DASH's (at approximately 27% of daily energy intake) as well as lower than the traditional Mediterranean (42%). About 7% of total energy intake still comes from saturated fat, as opposed to 6% for DASH and 9% for the Mediterranean. The highest intake of carbohydrate (58%) is still the total calories (versus 55% DASH and 42% Mediterranean). Protein intake remains between the lower Mediterranean (13%) and higher DASH (18%).

Overall, the commonalities of the above dietary patterns outweigh the differences. These include high intakes in unrefined sugars (mostly vegetables), moderate or high amounts of legumes, a focus on lean meats (lean meats) and healthy fat profiles (lower in saturated fat and higher in omega-3 and monounsaturated oil). This is believed to have contributed to low CVD rates, a lower risk of certain cancers and a decreased chance of diabetes and other chronic diseases.

High sodium content has been a common problem in East Asian diets. It is most evident in the Japanese diet, which includes a high intake of pickled vegetable, soy sauces, miso, and salt fish. Studies suggest a relationship between higher sodium intakes and higher rates of stomach cancer and cerebrovascular Disease. Okinawa's salt intake was lower than in Japan. However, it is still higher than Japan. The Okinawan food scene has a variety of dishes.

A strong influence of the Southeast Asian and southern Chinese cultures (bittergreens, spices peppers, and turmeric) is a reflection of their past participation in trade. This happened in Okinawa prefecture, which was an independent kingdom until 1879 and was known as the Kingdom of the Ryukyus. High sodium intake has partly reduced hypertensive symptoms. This is due to the increased need for sodium in hot, humid climates like Okinawa.

Indigenous Islanders' Diet

The islanders' traditional diet includes 30% green and white vegetables. Traditional Japanese food usually contains large amounts rice. The Okinawa diet, however, has smaller amounts. The Okinawa sweet potato is the mainstay. The Okinawan diet is 30% lower in sugar than the Japanese average and only 15% higher in grains.

Okinawan cooking uses smaller portions of green, yellow, and fish. There is also a smaller amount of rice in Okinawan than on mainland Japan. Many dishes are prepared with pork and fish in broth that includes a variety herbs and other ingredients. Satsuma sweet potato forms the center of Okinawa's diet. The sweet potato contributes to the island's self sufficiency. The Okinawa sweet Potato does not have a significant impact on blood sugar. Not only are the potatoes used, but the leaves also come from the plant. Miso soup uses the leaves often. The Okinawan bitter melons have been proven to have some antidiabetic qualities. Okinawa's bittermelon is called "Goyain" and is often served with the Okinawa national dish, "Goya Champuru". The bitter melon works in the same way as sweet potatoes to regulate blood sugar.

Traditional food also contains a small amount (less than half a cup per day) of fish and more in the form of soy and other legumes (6% of total calories). Pork is highly sought after, but only a few people eat it. Every part of the pork is edible, even its internal organs.

A comparison of Okinawa's sample, which had the longest life expectancy at 65 years old, with a sample from Akita Prefecture which had shorter life expectancies, revealed that Okinawa received significantly more calcium, vitamin A, B1, B2, C and higher amounts of energy from protein and fats than Akita. Akita had lower salt intake than Okinawa.

Okinawa still has a lower pork consumption per head (3g per day), than the Japanese national median. For example, in Okinawa in 1979, the annual average for pork consumption was 7.9 kilograms (17 lb). This exceeded the Japanese national standard by approximately 50%. Healthy everyday foodstuffs for pigs include their feet, ears, and stomach.

Okinawans' dietary intake is lower than that of other Japanese circa 1950. Short summary: The Okinawans in 1950 consumed sweet potatoes for 849g out of 1262 grams of food, 69% of their total calories.

Aside from their long lives expectancy, islanders are also known for their low mortality rate from certain types and cardiovascular disease. Wilcox, 2007, compared the age-adjusted deaths of Okinawans to those of Americans. They found that in 1995, an Okinawan was 8x less likely than Americans to die due to coronary heart disease. 7x less likely were Americans to die because of prostate cancer. 6.5x less likely were Americans to die as a result of breast cancer. 2.5x less likely were Americans to die from colon and stomach cancer.

The Okinawan-style diet described above was common on the islands right up until the 1960s. The diet has shifted to Western and Japanese traditions, with fat intake increasing from about 6% up to 27% of total caloric intake, and sweet potatoes being replaced by rice or bread.

This shift has led to a decline in longevity. Okinawans live longer than the Japanese.

Okinawa also has seaweed, especially konbu (or kombu). This is a low-calorie food option. The plant is rich with protein, amino acids, and minerals, such as iodine, just like the rest of the island's greenery. Wawakame is another popular seaweed. Like konbu wakame contains minerals such as calcium, magnesium, and Iodine. Seaweed and tofu are consumed daily in various forms. Kazuhiko Tarai, a gerontologist, stated that Okinawa's most used cooking fat is monounsaturated fat - lard. Although it's often called a "saturated" fat, lard contains 50 percent monounsaturated and 40 percent saturated fats. It also has 10 percent polyunsaturated. Taira says that Okinawans consume 100 grams of fish and pork each day to maintain their health.

Turmeric is a common ingredient in the Okinawan Diet. It has been widely used throughout history, especially in South Asia, for its supposed health benefits. The Okinawan use turmeric in tea and spice.

Okinawaans can enjoy many benefits from this diet. These include weight loss with age, a low BMI and low risk for age-related illnesses. This diet is good for fighting disease. As we mentioned, the diet contains many ingredients that are believed to have antioxidant and anti-aging properties. Science has never shown any ingredient or food to have anti-aging abilities. The Okinawa diet has 100 ingredients that have been tested and found to be anti-obese.

The diet contains similar foods as the traditional Okinawan diet, but has a higher energy intake. The primary focus of this diet is to determine the food energy density of every food item.

According to this diet, food can be divided into four categories according to caloric densities. The "featherweight," foods with less than 0.8 calories pergram (3.3kJ/g), can be eaten without any concern. The "lightweight" foods have a caloric density of 1.5 to 3.0 cal per gram and should be consumed in moderation. The middleweight foods, with a caloric density between 1.5 to 3.0 cal per gram, should also be eaten moderately. Finally, one should limit one's intake of the "heavyweight" foods which contain 3 to 9 calorie per gram.

"FUNCTIONAL FOODS" IN THE TRADITIONAL OKINAWAN DIET

It has received increasing attention from health-promoting elements of the Okinawan traditional diet. Numerous studies have been undertaken to examine the individual components of the diet, as well as how they impact health status in vitro, in live animals, and in human clinical trials. Okinawa's cuisine blurs the lines between medicine (food) and medicine (herbs such as fuchiba/mugwort, sweet potato leaf, ichoba/fennel), ichoba/fennel), and green seaweed), as well as other foods that are both used for medicine and food. All of them contain powerful antioxidants. For example, aasa Seaweed contains nearly 9000 mg of Carotene per 100g. Although space is limited, this brief review will cover some of the interesting work. We chose

The traditional Okinawan diet has low-GI 'functional foods'. These foods are low in caloric density but high in nutrients and are being researched for their health benefits.

such as CVD or cancer.

Flavonoid Rich Tofu, Other Soy Foods

The Okinawan tradition has a high amount of legumes. Soy products are a major component of the Okinawan's longevity and health. The main source for protein was soy, which is why older Okinawans seem to have consumed more soy in the forms of miso soup, tofu, and other varieties than other people. We found that they consume on average three ounces of soy products each day, mainly in the form tofu and miso (soy sauce). Flavonoids in soybeans are known to have antioxidant-like benefits and other health-promoting properties. Okinawa's tofu contains less water than the Japanese, but is higher in healthy fats and proteins. This not only improves the flavor, but also increases isoflavone levels. This may possibly be due to

Okinawa's extremely low rates for breast and prostate carcinoma.

Potential Health Benefits

Clinical studies have shown that intake of soy proteins can lower CVD risk factors. This resulted in U.S. Food and Drug Administration approval in 1999 of the food labeling health claim for soy proteins in prevention of coronary disease. A meta-analysis of randomized controlled trials has shown that soyisoflavones can reduce serum total cholesterol in humans. There is limited evidence that soy isoflavones can also be used to treat other health conditions, such as menopausal symptoms, and the ability to slow down postmenopausal bone losses. However, these findings are encouraging. It is interesting to note that Japan has high soy consumption and that women there have less problems during menopause than in Western countries. Also, their death rates from breast or hormone dependent cancers are lower than those of Westerners. Despite encouraging ecological evidence, as well as the generally positive results of observational and epidemiological research indicating that soy consumption reduces breast cancer risks in women, we are still studying the safety and efficacy for treating or preventing cancer of the breast, prostate, and endometrium. While more evidence is needed, we are still waiting.

Soy isoflavones. There is strong consensus that soy foods may be beneficial for your cardiovascular and overall health. They are high in polyunsaturated and fiber fats, vitamins, minerals, and low amounts of saturated fat. Recent laboratory research has shown that enzymes derived from fermented soy, or natto, may prevent the accumulation of certain plaques in brains linked to Alzheimer's. Soy also has a low GI.

You can regulate insulin and blood sugar levels.

Goya (Momordica charantia)

Okinawa's bittermelon is called "Goya" in Okinawa. Goya is a gourd with a distinctive appearance. It looks similar to a cucumber, but has rough, pockmarked flesh. Okinawan cuisine's mainstay is Goya. It's used in salads (raw and cooked), stir-fried, sandwiches and tempura. You can also find it in juice and tea. Fast food restaurants even sell goya burgers or goya rings. Goya, which is a member in the melon group, probably came to Okinawa via trade between ancient China and the Ming- and Manchu dynasties. It is available in North America at Asian food stores and Chinese markets.

Potential Health Benefits

Goya, which is low in calories, high in fiber, and rich in vitamin C, has been used to treat various ailments in India and South America. Folk medicinal uses include laxatives and tonics as well as laxatives and laxatives. Alternate therapies include bitter melon, which is used to lower blood glucose in diabetics mellitus patients. Charantin and vicine have anti-diabetic qualities.

polypeptide p, and other bioactive ingredients such as antioxidants. Although bitter gourd extracts have shown hypoglycemic as well as metabolic effects in cell cultures and animal and human studies, the mechanism for action, including regulation of insulin or altered glucose metabolism and its insulin like effect, remains a mystery. In vitro evidence has also shown antiviral and anticancer properties, including the human immunodeficiencyvirus. Bitter melon should only be used in well-powered, randomized, placebo-controlled trials to ensure safety and efficacy.

Konnyaku (Amorphophallus konjac)

Konnyaku is Japanese traditional jelly made with a yamlike tuber called devil's tongue. It originated in China and Indochina. It is an ancient food. References to it are found in the Wamyouruijou Japanese dictionary which was first published around 1100 years ago (930 a.d.). Konnyaku lacks flavor, but it easily absorbs other flavors when cooked. Konnyaku jelly has been made with the flour derived from this Japanese roots. You can get it in different sizes: as a dense, dense, and gelatinous cake or as thin noodles. Okinawans attribute konnyaku's high fiber content to the fact that it "cleanses your stomach.

Potential Health Benefits

Konnyaku is very low in calories and high in fiber and vitamin C, making it ideal for weight control. Konnyaku is over 90% water. The remainder is glucomannan. Konnyaku can be used as an adjunct therapy to high cholesterol and type 2.

Diabetes because of its positive effects in blood sugar

Shiitake Mushrooms (Lentinus.edodes).

The shiitake, a large, dark brown and umbrella-shaped mushroom, has been used for centuries by Asian cultures. Shiitake mushrooms are still an important dietary staple in some countries.

China and were once important sources of protein in Japan and other East Asian countries. They are often dried in Okinawa and wrapped in beautiful gift bags. Dry shiitake mushroom are a great ingredient for low-fat, high-calorie healthy dishes.

Senior Americans eat healthier diets

Potential Health Benefits

Shiitake mushrooms may have immunomodulatory and lipidlowering properties. They also appear to be antitumor and other beneficial or therapeutic benefits. One of the components of shiitake mushrooms, lentinan, is a polysaccharide. Japan has approved intravenous lentinan, a highly purified and effective anticancer drug, for patients suffering from stomach or pancreatic carcinoma. Because of their potential usefulness in preventing or treating serious health conditions such as cancer and hypercholesterolemia, functional mushrooms deserve

You will need to do a more thorough investigation.

Gobo (Arctium lappa)

Burdock, or gobo, is a short root vegetable that has a dark brown skin and grayish-white pulp. It is rich in iron with a sweet, earthy aroma. It is also a common folk medicine in Okinawa (and many other parts the world), and it is well-known as a 'blood purifier''.

Potential Health Benefits

Burdock root, although low in calories, is high in inulin. Also, it is rich in two types fiber: inulin (a type of inulin) and mucilage (a type of spongy fiber). This thick, glutinous substance is related to the natural sugars and used in medicine and as an emollient. Inulin, an edible burdock root, has been found to have probiotic properties. This could increase health by improving your health.

Beneficial bacteria in the stomach. These properties may be responsible for burdock's purported soothing effect on the digestive tract. Its high fiber level is why burdock is so popular in Korea. In Korea, raw burdock are cut into thin strips and marinated before being eaten.

While the efficacy and safety of the "burdock vinegar diet" has yet to be proven, the positive effects of fiber on weightloss are well documented. Animal studies have also shown that burdock reduces liver damage. Burdock might play an important role in protecting the liver.

Hechima (Luffa cylindrica)

Hechima, one of the gourd families, was introduced to Okinawa 3 centuries ago. It is closely associated with Luffa actionangulla, which is also eaten in Hawaii, and parts of Southeast Asia. While hechima is not eaten much in Japan, mainland Japanese people do eat it. They do however use the dry outer core to make a dish scrubber and body. It is a low-calorie vegetable, high in vitamin A, folate, carotenoids and other interesting proteins, which could have significant health effects.

Potential Health Benefits

Folkloric health claims concerning hechima are based on its potential to prevent cancer and boost the immune system. Cucurbitaceae plants may have one or more of eight proteins found in extracts. These include anticancer, antiviral and immune-enhancing properties. There have been over 20 studies on hechima's special proteins, known as luffin-proteins.

Seaweeds

Seaweeds have long been a staple food in Okinawa Japan, China, Japan, and other parts Asia. "Seaweed" can be loosely defined as multicellular, macro-scicular marine algae. Red, brown and green algae are all included in the term. The Okinawan culinary staple is made up of more than 12 varieties. It is possible that seaweeds could have medicinal properties. Some have been used to treat illnesses like arthritis, flu and cancer. However most of these claims still need to be proven in clinical trials.

Okinawan cuisine consists mainly of wakame, mozuku and wakame. Kombu is one the main ingredients for dashi (soup) broth. Mozuku is another brown seaweed enjoyed throughout Japan. It is easily farmed in Okinawa, where it is simply done by placing the mozuku on a net and then spreading that net over the coral reef. It is eaten mostly with vinegar, in noodle dishes and with rice or jelly. Wakame, a kelp with a blackish color and mild flavor, is soaked to turn green. Okinawa tradition calls for it to be added to miso soup together with tofu. Hijiki is a dark-colored vegetable with a bittersweet flavor. It is sold in strips of match-size length. It is delicious when it is simmered with whole soybeans, vegetables, and okara. Aasa or laver is a yellow-green algae that grows on rocks on Okinawan beaches. Okinawa has a lot to offer in terms of weekend activities, such as collecting seaweed and storing it for later use in soups or tempura dishes.

Potential Health Benefits

Seaweeds offer a very low caloric density, are extremely nutrient-dense and high levels of protein, ioine and folate. They also have significant antioxidant abilities. They offer a wealth of therapeutic options and nutraceuticals that are still in development. A seaweed carotenoid called fucoxanthin has been proven to have many beneficial effects on metabolism. In animal models it was shown that it significantly reduced blood glucose and plasma levels as well as increasing the level in hepatic hexaenoic and attenuating weight gains.

Intervention for metabolic disorder. Astaxanthin (a xanthophyll xanthophyll cotenoid) is a powerful and broad-ranging antioxidant that can be obtained from microalgae. It also occurs naturally within a variety of living organisms including fungi as well as complex plants and crustaceans. Results from multiple species support the antioxidant/anti-inflammatory properties of astaxanthin as a novel potential candidate for development as a therapeutic agent for cardiovascular oxidative stress and inflammation. Fucoidan is an sulfated polysaccharide that can be found in brown seaweeds like wakame or mozuku. Research on fucoidan continues to focus on two main forms: Ffucoidan which is.95% comprised of sulfated ester of fucose; and Ufucoidan which contains approximately 20% of glucuronic acid. Ffucoidan (and U-fucoidan) are both nutraceuticals. It could also be thought to have anticancer effects. Japanese researchers discovered that Fucoidan can incite apoptosis within human lymphoma cell line cells. Additional studies have also demonstrated it can inhibit hyperplasia among animal models. Potentially antithrombotic agents can also be found in the algal and invertebrate Polysaccharides.

TRADITIONAL SPICES and HERBS

Even though the USDA recommends that you reduce fat, salt, sugar, and other unhealthy substances from your diet, it's extremely difficult for most people. All three add flavor and/or texture. The herbs and spices are a substitute. The Okinawans are fondly familiar with many herbs, spices, flavors, and flavourings that they use in their cooking. These not only add a rich flavor to the food, but also provide medicinal properties. Many have been used in Ayurvedic medicine and traditional Chinese medicine for many years. Many traditional herbs, spices, and spices contain phytochemicals. These herbs and spices claim many health benefits, but most have been drawn from Okinawan traditional medicine practices and are not yet tested. The health benefits of other herbs and spices have been demonstrated in the lab and even clinical trials. Below are some of our favorite herbs and spices.

Ucchin (Curcuma longa)

Turmeric (or ucchin) is a herb that every Okinawan is familiar with. While many people consume it as a tea or take it in tablet format to "strengthen liver", particularly when drinking alcohol (for prevention of hangovers), most people use it as a spice for soups and curries. It has many uses.

Curcumin, which gives yellow curries a distinctive orange-yellow shade, is responsible for their unique color. Originating in India, turmeric belonged to the ginger tribe and was probably brought to Okinawa through the spice trade. Ayurvedic medicine employs turmeric for a wide range of conditions, including skin, respiratory, and gastrointestinal, as well pain, wounds, liver disorders, and other ailments. Turmeric has become just as vital to Okinawan cuisines and apothecaries as it has in India. Let's take a look at its potential health benefits to see why.

Potential Health Benefits

Turmeric has long been revered for its folk healing properties, especially by traditional healers. In India, researchers later confirmed that it has significant antiinflammatory properties. Turmeric is also known to have significant antimicrobial capabilities, which is one of the reasons it has been used for centuries as a treatment for wounds and pain. Studies have shown that Turmeric is as effective at treating pain associated with rheumatologic diseases such as osteoarthritis and rheumatoid arthritis (NSAIDs), as well as postoperative pain.

pain. Turmeric seems to be able even to protect the stomach's protective mucosal surface against NSAIDs. NSAIDs have a reputation for promoting bleeding.

Other potential benefits of turmeric have been reported. These include significant antioxidant capacity, which may be linked to its anticancer properties. Turmeric has been shown to be an inhibitor of cancer cell growth in vitro and vivo. Curcumin's ability to impact multiple targets is evident in its activity against leukemia and lymphoma as well as gastrointestinal and genitourinary tumors, breast and ovarian cancers, genitourinary and genitourinary carcinomas, genitourinary and gastrointestinal cancers, sarcoma, and head and neck cancer squamous cell carcinoma. The promise of turmeric for chronic diseases is not limited to cancer. Dietary components of turmeric, such as curcumin, which inhibits inflammation and amyloid beta oligomerization and consequently increases apoptosis, are of particular interest with respect to chronic inflammatory response, brain injury, and beta-amyloid-associated pathology in Alzheimer's disease; curcumin has emerged as a candidate

This is important. Curcumin acts not only as an antioxidant, but also stimulates the heat shock response. The use of curcumin in food supplements is being investigated as a new nutritional approach to reduce amyloid pathology and oxidative damages in Alzheimer's disease. The safety and efficacy in turmeric for medical purposes still need to be confirmed using placebo-controlled, interventional trials. However, the preliminary evidence suggests that it may be worth considering for a variety of age-related diseases.

Fuchiba (Artemisia vulgaris)

In Okinawa's past, fuchiba had been the only treatment available for stomach disorders. Fuchiba is commonly known in the West as mugwort. It can be purchased in teaform or liquid form, and also dried for use in cooking. Mugwort is used in Okinawan cookery in vegetable pilafs and soups. It has dark green leaves that smell a bit like rosemary. Mugwort can be used to help upset stomachs. It also acts as an herbal remedy for strengthening the liver. Both claims require more scientific testing.

Potential Health Benefits

Fuchiba's levels of carotene are very high (upwards of 9000 mg/100g). Folkloric claims include the ability to treat multiple conditions, including gout or gallstones, respiratoryailments, gallstones and kidney stones, and infections.

Gastritis, tuberculosis, wounds and others are all possible. Rootsfrom mugwort appear to have sedative effects; they are usedin traditional Chinese medicine to treat neuroses, depression,irritability, restlessness, insomnia, and anxiety. Mulgwort has been the topic of over 100 studies. Many of these studies support its folk uses. Artemisia is a traditional stomach protector that was tested against ethanol-induced gastric cancer in rats.

Artemisia is used to treat malaria and other infectious diseases. Chemicallyactive components are found in its seeds, fresh roots, andleaves that are in the same class of compounds--flavonoids--as are found in ginkgo biloba, green tea, and soy andsoy products. Animal studies with the aqueous extract ofArtemisia vulgaris resultedin a significant rise in blood glutathione levels and superoxide demutase activities.

Aqueous Artemisia vulgaris extracts may be an effective source of natural antioxidants. This is evident from the high serum levelsof ascorbic Acid.

Hihatsu (Piper hancei)

The Okinawan Pepper can be dried, ground and sprinkled on food. This pepper is an important ingredient in hot and spicy Okinawa dishes. The leaves of this plant are used in tempura recipes, and can often be found in the apothecaries at Okinawan herbalists.

Potential Health Benefits

Hihatsu, an Okinawan herbal remedy, has been used to treat stomach disorders and gout. Ayurvedic medicine has used hihatsu to treat stomach issues and gout. Hot peppersare a good source of dietary antioxidants, encompassing, inaddition to widespread compounds (flavonoids, phenolic acids,carotenoids, vitamin A, ascorbic acid, tocopherols), morespecific constituents, such as the pungent capsaicinoids(capsaicin, dihydrocapsaicin, and related analogues), whichhave shown remarkable antioxidant activity and the ability toprotect linoleic acid against free radical attack in simple invitro systems, inhibiting both its auto-oxidation and its iron- orethylenediaminetetraacetic acid-mediated oxidation.

A CULTURAL MODEL HEALTHYEATING TO HEALTHY AGEING

Improving Cardiovascular Health

CVD, principally coronary heart disease andstroke, are the most common causes of death in North America. The majority of Americans over 65 experience arterial stiffening, which is a major risk factor for stroke, coronary artery disease. Heart attack, heart failure and dementia are all possible. CVD risk factors are those that indicate the health of thearteries. These include cholesterol levels, homocysteine level, blood pressure and oxidative stresses.

Here are some foods in the Okinawan Diet that you might like

This contributes to reduced cardiovascular risk factors

Vegetables, legumes, and other phytonutrient-rich food are all examples. Asdiscussed previously, these foods contain properties that areproving to be important to heart health such as the antioxidantvitamins A, C, and E, anthocyanins and other polyphenols,carotenoids, flavonoids, and more. A recent study on the antioxidant activityof Okinawa vegetables revealed a high level of phenolic chemicals and strong radicalscavenging actions in traditional Okinawan vegetables. Carotenoids are most abundant in brightly colored orange, yellow, or green vegetables in Okinawa. The best-known carotenoids include the betacarotene in carrots as well as orange sweetpotatoes. Lycopene is found in tomatoes and watermelon. Flavonoids are plant compounds similar to hormones and antioxidants that exist in morethan 4000 varieties. They are found in onions, tomatoes, broccoli, red wine, green, black, and Oolong teas among otherfoods. Healthy omega-3 fat, found in fish and soy oil, is also animportant part of the Okinawan diet, and like the othercomponents mentioned, has been shown in well-conductedstudies to play an important role in cardiovascular health.

These food elements are essential to the diet.

Recent clinical trials that have been well-designed and conducted have demonstrated the effectiveness of reducing cardiovascular risk factors. It consisted of foods available in regular supermarkets,including common vegetables consumed in Okinawa, such asbroccoli, carrots, red peppers, tomatoes, onions, cauliflower,okra, and eggplant. Other functional foods were wholegrains such oats or barley, vegetable margarine, almonds and soy protein products such as soymilk and soysausages as well as soy cold cuttings and soy burgers.

These phytonutrient-rich foods that are high in fiber and healthier oils, like soy, reduce LDL cholesterol by about 30%.

This suggests that LDL-lowering dietary strategies (e.g. fiber, flavonoids or vegetableprotein) can have additive effects when incorporated in a healthy diet. This approach was equally effective as statins. They have been the standard therapy for high cholesterol for many decades. It also offered many other benefits such as weight loss and lower inflammation (Creactive protein levels).

Similar risk factors to diabetes and CVD were also lower.

Walford et al. The Biosphere 2 Study was initiated when subjects were given a diet that was "calorically restricted" in the first six months. This diet was very similar to the Okinawan tradition. Average bodyweight loss of male subjects was 18%; women experienced a decrease of 10%. Blood pressure fell 20% onaverage. On average, diabetes indicators such as blood glucose or insulin levels fell 30%. Meanwhile, cholesterol levels dropped from 195 averaging to 125.

Todoriki led the local research team.

The "Champuru Studies" team have been performingclinical interventions using

Okinawan vegetable such as goya ("Momordicacharantia"), green papaya ("Carica papaya"), handama ("Gynurabicolor"), karashina ("Brassicajuncea"), fuchiba ("Artemisiavulgaris") and fundanso ("Betavulgaris") in an effort to investigate thehealth-promoting qualities of the traditional diet in a evidence-based research. Results so farhave been impressive and have revealed that increasingconsumption of such vegetables, commonly consumed in thetraditional dietary pattern, can increase potassium excretion in normotensive healthy young women as well as raiselevels of circulating endothelial progenitor cells.

As well as being associated with atherosclerotic risk factors, circulating endothelialprogenitor cell activity is believed to play an important rolein maintaining the integrity of vascular vessel walls. As such, the changes in the endothelialprogenitorcells in these young women wereinversely associated with both changes in total cholesterol and LDL cholesterol. We also noticed an increase in serum folicacid and a decrease in plasma homocysteine.

Lower risk of chronic diseases

Okinawans are not only long-lived but also have fewer chronic conditions such as diabetes and heart disease.

Okinawan foods have essential nutrients, fiber, antioxidants, and anti-inflammatory substances. However, they are low on calories, refined sugar, saturated fats, and calories.

Sweet potatoes account for the bulk of calories in the traditional diet. Some experts claim that the sweet potato may be one of your healthiest food choices.

Sweet potatoes have a healthy supply of fiber and a low glycemic [GI], which means they don't contribute to rapid rises or spikes in blood glucose. They are also rich in vitamins A, B, and C, which is essential for their nutritional value.

The powerful plant compounds carotenoids found in sweet potatoes, and other colorful vegetables are also present on Okinawa.

Carotenoids provide antioxidant and anti-inflammatory benefits. They may also play a role preventing type 2 diabetes and heart disease.

The Okinawa diet also contains a lot of soy.

Research has shown that soy-based foods can be associated with lower rates of certain chronic illnesses, such as heart disease, and certain types cancers like breast cancer.

Okinawa diet: Possible downsides

While the Okinawa diet offers many benefits, there are still some potential drawbacks.

Fairly restrictive

The traditional Okinawa diet does not include certain food groups, but many of these foods are quite healthy.

This can make it hard to stick to a diet and limit important nutrients. It is possible that certain Okinawan dishes may not be easily accessible, depending on where you are located.

The diet has very little dairy, fruits, nuts and seeds. These foods can provide a rich source of vitamins, minerals and antioxidants which can help improve your health.

You don't have to restrict these food groups. However, it could be harmful if you fail to replenish nutrients.

People prefer the Okinawa mainstream version for weight loss because it offers more options in food.

Potentiation for high sodium

The Okinawa diet's biggest drawback may be the high sodium content.

Some versions of this diet allow for 3,200 mg per day. This amount of sodium may not be appropriate for all people, especially those with high bloodpressure.

The American Heart Association recommends limiting your sodium intake to 1,500mg daily if high blood pressure exists, and 2,300mg daily if normal blood pressure.

High sodium intake can result in increased blood pressure.

Notably, the Okinawa Diet is high in potassium. This may help offset some of the possible negative effects of high sodium intake. Your kidneys will remove excess fluid from your body, which results in lower blood pressure.

If you're interested to try the Okinawa lifestyle but need to be careful about sodium, it is best to stay away from foods high in sodium like miso or dashi.

Is Okinawa the right diet for you?

Even though the Okinawa Diet has many health benefits, some people may prefer a more restricted or low-carb diet.

It may have several benefits, such as the emphasis on vegetables, fiber, antioxidant-rich foods, and a restriction on sugar, refined grain, and excess fat.

Lifestyle principles that Okinawan culture promotes, such as daily exercise and mindfulness, could also have health benefits.

These principles can, however, be applied to many other types of diets and lifestyles.

If you're not sure if the Okinawa lifestyle is right for your diet, talk to your physician or dietitian about creating a customized plan.

TOFU CHAMPURU

Serves: 2

Prep Time: 10 Mins

Cook Time: 20 Minutes

Total time: 30 minutes

INGREDIENTS

- 1 momen-tofu

1/4 onion

1 bunch Chinese Chives

1 tablespoon sesame oils

1 tablespoon bonito powder

1/4 teaspoon sake

- 1/4 tsp soy sauce

1/4 tsp salt

1 Liter of water

DIRECTIONS

1. Cut the tofu in 10-12 pieces

2. Place the tofu in boiling water and boil for 2-3 min

3. Cut thin slices of the Chinese chives (onion and Chinese chives)

4. In a frying skillet, stir-fry tofu in sesame oils

5. Add onions, bonito flakes, onion, and Chinese chillies

6. Serve when you're ready

PAPAYA CHAMPURU

Serves: 4

Prep Time: 10 minutes

Cook Time: 30 Minutes

Total time: 40 minutes

INGREDIENTS

- 1/4 papaya

1/2 carrot

- 1 green peppers

Chinese chives - 14 pound

- 2 oz. Spam

- 1 tsp dashi stock granules

- 1 tsp soy sauce

- 1 oz. lard

DIRECTIONS

1. Slice the papaya in thin strips

2. Julienne the green and yellow carrots

3. The Chinese chives can be curtailed and the spam cut into strips

4. In a skillet melt the butter and stir fry the vegetables

5. Continue to stir fry the rest of the ingredients.

6. Add Chinese chives, soy sauce and dashi soup to your dish

7. Cook until well done. Transfer to a plate.

INAMURUCHI

Serves: 4

Prep Time: 10 Mins

Cook Time: 30 Minutes

Total time: 40 minutes

INGREDIENTS

- 1 lb. pork

- 4 pieces mushrooms

- 1/4 lb. Kasutera Kamaboko

- 1/2 lb. Inamuruchi konjac

4 tablespoons Inamuruchi mayo

- 1 pack bonito powder

- 1 Liter water

DIRECTIONS

1. Boil the pork until it becomes soft

2. Put the mushrooms in warm water.

3. Cut the ingredients into thin slices

4. Boil the water until it is 1L. Add 1 packet of bonito powder and heat for 4-5 minutes

5. Put the pork pieces in a pan and cook for 12 to 11 minutes

6. When ready, add Inamuruchi sour cream and serve

RAFUTE

Serves: 4

Prep time: 10 Minutes

Cook Time: 45 Mins

Total Time: 55 Minutes

INGREDIENTS

- 1 lb. Pork belly

- 1 lb. daikon radish

1 tablespoon rice

1/4 cup sake

- 2 tablespoons soy sauce

1 Tablespoon Mirin

1 tablespoon sugar

- 1-piece ginger

- Green shallots

DIRECTIONS

1. Cut Daikon Radishes into thick cubes

2. Put the pork into a pressure cooker. Add water. Rice and cook on low for about 15-20 minutes

3. You can take everything out of your pressure cooker

4. In a second pot, combine sake, mirin dark muscovado, mirin, mirin, and ginger

5. Mix the pork and daikon with radish in a saucepan. Simmer for 20 minutes

6. After heat has been turned off, add green shallots.

ASA SOUP

Serves: 4

Prep Time: 10 Mins

Cook Time: 20 Minutes

Total time: 30 minutes

INGREDIENTS

Dry Asaa - 12g

1/4 block tofu

600 cc soup bonito

- Soy sauce

DIRECTIONS

1. Asa in warm water. Boil the soup.

2. Add small cubes tofu to the mixture and mix well

3. Add soy sauce to the pot and continue cooking

4. Once you're ready, take off the heat.

SQUID INK NOODLE SOUP

Serves: 4

Prep time: 10 Minutes

Cook Time: 20 Minutes

Total time: 30 minutes

INGREDIENTS

- 2 lbs. udon noodles

- 1 acorn squash

1 tablespoon olive Oil

- 5 cups chicken broth

2 packages of squidink

1 carrot

DIRECTIONS

1. Put the noodles in a saucepan and heat.

2. Cook the squash in a pot. Once it is browned, add the broth.

3. Mix the broth with the squid, ink, and cook until thickened.

4. Cook the carrot in a separate pan for another 3-4 mins

5. Serve soup, noodles, and milk in a bowl

JAPANESE STEWED ROCKFISH

Serves: 2

Prep Time: 10 Mins

Cook Time: 20 Minutes

Total time: 30 minutes

INGREDIENTS

- 2 rockfish (Mebaru).

250 ml Water

150ml sake

- 2 tablespoons soy sauce

2 tablespoons mirin

2 tsp sugar

DIRECTIONS

1. Put mirin and soy sauce in a pot. Add sugar, water, salt, and sake to the pot. Bring it to a boil.

2. Add fish to the pot and bring it to a boil

3. Once your dish is ready to serve, place it on a plate and enjoy

NINJIN SHIRISHIRI

Serves: 2

Prep time: 10 Minutes

Cook Time: 20 Minutes

Total time: 30 minutes

INGREDIENTS

1 carrot

- 2 oz. tuna

- 1 egg

1 tsp sesame Oil

- 1/4 tsp soy sauce

2 tablespoons bonito powder

DIRECTIONS

1. Chop the carrot into thin strips and grate.

2. Cook the tuna in sesame and vegetable oil. Add water to the pan.

3. Sprinkle with salt and season with soy sauce

4. Salt and egg are added to the egg. Beat it until smooth

5. Heat until bonito Flakes are added.

6. Place the ninjinshihiri on top of a plate.

PORK TAMAGO ONIGIRI

Serves: 6

Prep Time: 5 Mins

Cook Time: 10 Minutes

Total time: 15 minutes

INGREDIENTS

- 3 oz. dried kelp

Spam in 1/4 can

- 3 eggs

- 1/2 lb. rice

- 6 pieces roasted laver

DIRECTIONS

1. Put the eggs in a skillet and cook until golden brown.

2. Slice spam in six portions

3. Spread rice over the laver

4. Mix pork, egg and cheese on top. Fold.

5. Serve when ready

JIMAMIMI DOFU WITH PEANUTS

Serves: 4

Prep time: 10 Minutes

Cook Time: 30 minutes

Total time: 40 minutes

INGREDIENTS

- 1/2 lb. peanuts

- 2 oz. katakuriko

1 Liter of water

- 2 tablespoons dashi stock

1 tablespoon soy sauce

1 Tablespoon Mirin

- 1-piece ginger

DIRECTIONS

1. Let peanuts soak in water

2. Blend the peanuts till smooth

3. Place the contents of your blender in a pan, add katakuriko, and heat on low heat.

4. Line a mold, then pour the mixture into it

5. Cover the mixture and let it chill in cold water

NAKAMI SOUP

Serves: 4

Prep Time: 10 Mins

Cook Time: 60 Mins

Total time: 70 minutes

INGREDIENTS

- 1 lb. PORK GUTTER

- 1/2 lb. pork

- 4 mushrooms

- 1/4 kamaboko fish paste

- 1 pack konnyaku

- 1 L soup stock

1 tsp salt

1 tablespoon soy sauce

- Wheat flour

DIRECTIONS

1. Make thin strips from the kamaboko (pork, mushrooms)

2. Boil the pork bones for 10 minutes

3. Mix the pork and wheat flour in a bowl.

4. Put the mushroom, water, and dashi soup in a saucepan. Heat for 45-50min

5. Serve with soy sauce.

TACO ROICE

Serves: 2

Prep time: 10 Minutes

Cook Time: 30 Minutes

Total Time: 40 minutes

INGREDIENTS

2 cups cooked rice

1 tablespoon olive Oil

1/4 onion

1 clove garlic

1 pinch black pepper

1/4 chili powder

1/2 lb. Ground beef

1/4 tablespoon soya sauce

1/4 teaspoon sake

DIRECTIONS

1. Prepare the rice before you begin.

2. Cook the onion, garlic, and olive oil in a large skillet until soft.

3. Mix together pepper, chili powder, and salt.

4. Mix in the beef and cook it until the meat is tender.

5. Add soy sauce, sake, and mix well

6. When you are done, add lettuce, tomato, and serve

GOYA CHAMPURU

Serves: 3

Prep Time: 10 Mins

Cook Time: 40 Mins

Total Time:50Minutes

INGREDIENTS

1 oz. 1 oz.

1 oz. soy sauce

1 Tablespoon stock

1 teaspoon salt

1 oz. mirin

1 tablespoon sesame oils

1 goya

1/2 lb. bacon

2 eggs

1 tofu

DIRECTIONS

1. Combine mirin, soy sauces, stock and salt in a bowl. Mix well. Set the sauce aside

2. Slice the goya in half. Scoop the seeds out

3. Cut goya into pieces and soak for at least 10-15 minutes in warm water.

4. Reduce the bacon into small strips and sprinkle with salt.

5. Cut the tofu cubes

6. Place olive oil in a pan and heat until the olive oil is melted.

7. Mix in sesame, bacon, and goya.

8. Mix the eggs well and add the eggs to the pan.

9. Ready to serve with goyachanpuru

FAJITA & CHICKEN TACOS

Serves: 2

Prep Time: 5 Mins

Cook Time: 15 Mins

Total Time: 20 Minutes

INGREDIENTS

4 corn tortillas

2 fajitas

1 chicken breast

1/4 onion

1/4 green bell Pepper

1 pinch pepper

1/2 lime

DIRECTIONS

1. Fry the fajitas.

2. Mix the chicken breast with the mixture.

3. While the chicken breasts are being cooked, you can add onion to the pan and pepper.

4. After mixing, add the mixture to corn tortillas. Add lime juice and then serve.

STIR-FRIED GOYA

Serves: 2

Prep Time: 5 Mins

Cook Time: 15 Mins

Total Time:20 minutes

INGREDIENTS

1/4 Goya

1/2 lb. Tofu

1/4 lb. Pork

1/4 onion

1/2 carrot

2 beaten eggs

SEASONING

1 Tablespoon sake

1 tablespoon soya sauce

1 tablespoon oyster Sauce

1 tablespoon vegetable oil

1 tablespoon sesame oils

DIRECTIONS

1. Salt the goya and rinse it off.

2. Cook the tofu in a large skillet until it is browned.

3. Place the tofu in a pan.

4. Heat sesame oils, add the carrots, onions, goya, and pork. Stir for about 2-3 minutes

5. Combine tofu with seasoning. Stir until combined

6. Mix the beaten eggs well with the flour.

7. Season with salt, and serve when ready

CHICKEN TAQUITOS

Serves: 6

Prep Time: 15 Mins

Cook Time: 20 Minutes

Total Time: 35 minutes

INGREDIENTS

5-6 flour tortillas

2 lbs. Breast of chicken

1/4 cup cheddar cheese

1/4 cup Mexican mix

1 package taco rice

1 package of seasoning mix for fajitas

Season 1 tablespoon taco seasoning

1 tsp salt

DIRECTIONS

1. Preheat the oven to 325 F

2. Cook the rice in the meantime and then set it aside

3. Place bacon strips in a frying skillet and cook at low heat.

4. Mix in the fajita seasoning and chicken. Cook the rice for another 4-5 mins

5. Add salt and taco seasoning to the mixture. Mix well

6. To make tortilla wraps, add 2-3 spoons of Mexican mix to each wrap. Then sprinkle Mexican blend on top.

7. Toss the tortilla with cheese, and bake in the oven 12-15 minutes

8. When ready, take out and serve

TACO CASSEROLE

Serves: 5-6

Prep Time: 15 Mins

Cook Time: 30 minutes

Total Time: 45 minutes

INGREDIENTS

2 lb. Beef

1 onion

1 zucchini

2 cups of corn

1 can beans

1 package taco seasoning

Salt

4-5 cups cooked rice

Shredded Cheese

DIRECTIONS

1. In a frying skillet brown the beef. Then add the onion, zucchini, and continue to cook until it becomes tender.

2. Mix in taco seasonings, beans corn and tomatoes

3. Put 2 cups rice in each pan.

4. Serve the meat mixture over rice. Sprinkle cheese on top

5. Bake for 20-30 Minutes at 350 F

6. When done, take out of the oven.

FISH-TACO BOWLS

Serves: 4

Prep Time: 15 Mins

Cook Time: 20 Minutes

Total Time: 35 minutes

INGREDIENTS

1 cup brown Rice

1 cup water

1 lb. mahi mahi

1/2 tsp chili powder

1 tsp smoked paprika

1/4 teaspoon salt

1 tablespoon Canola oil

1 avocado

1 tablespoon lime juice

1 cup cabbage

1 cup jicama

1 cup tomatoes

1 serving lime dressing

DIRECTIONS

1. Combine rice, water and cook on high for about 10-12 minutes.

2. In a bowl, combine the garlic powder with chili powder, salt, pepper, and paprika.

3. Mix spice blends on both sides.

4. Put the fish in a skillet.

5. Cook each side for approximately 4-5 minutes

6. Take out the lime dressing once it is ready and mix with your favorite sauce

RICE & BEAN BURRITOS

Serves: 6

Prep Time: 15 Mins

Cook Time: 25 Minutes

Total Time:40Minutes

INGREDIENTS

6 burrito tortillas

1 lb. 1 lb.

1 cup water

4 oz. 4 oz.

1 can red bean

12 oz. salsa

1 cup cheese

1 green onion

DIRECTIONS

1. Preheat the oven at 350 F

2. For 5-6 minutes, brown the beef in an oven-proof skillet

3. Boil water, rice, beans in a pot for 10-12 minute

4. Put the beef aside and add half a cup rice mixture, half of a cheese, and a half-cup of salsa. Mix well

5. Put half of the salsa in a baking pan

6. Place about 3/4 of the rice mixture in a tortilla and roll it up.

7. Place the tortilla upside down in the dish

8. Add the remaining salsa to the tortillas. Then sprinkle cheese on top

9. Bake for 20-30 minute. Once the time is up, take it out and add green onion.

PORK CHOP CASSEROLE

Serves: 3

Prep time: 15 Minutes

Cook Time: 35 Minutes

Total Time:50 Minutes

INGREDIENTS

4 pork chops

2 cans jalapeno Refried Beans

2 packages taco rice

1 package Mexican Shredded Cheese

DIRECTIONS

1. Preheat the oven to 375 F

2. In a casserole dish spread refried beans

3. Make pork chops and serve with beans.

4. Place cooked rice on top. Cover with aluminum foil

5. Cook for 15-20 minutes covered. Cook for another 12-15 mins uncovered

6. When the food is ready, take it off the heat.

SATA ANDAGI

Serves: 6-8

Prep time: 15 Minutes

Cook Time: 15 Mins

Total Time:30 Minutes

INGREDIENTS

3/4 lb. Flour

1/4 lb. 1/4 lb.

1 teaspoon baking powder

2 eggs

2 Tbsp vegetable oil

DIRECTIONS

1. Mix the eggs with sugar and olive oil in a large bowl.

2. Mix in flour, baking powder, salt and pepper.

3. Form small balls of dough and fry in a pan.

4. When ready, remove and serve

PADTHAI SOMEN CHANPURU

Serves: 2

Prep Time: 5 minutes

Cook Time: 25 Minutes

Total Time: 30Minutes

INGREDIENTS

2 bundles of somen noodles

1 bag bean sprouts

1/4 bunch garlic-chives

1/4 Japanese leek

1 cabbage

2 eggs

1 dash squid

8-10 peanuts

2 tablespoons chili sauce

1 dash soy sauce

1/4 clove garlic

DIRECTIONS

1. Boil the somen noodles, then drain.

2. In a pan, fry the eggs.

3. Stir-fry the garlic and leek until tender. Then add shrimp, pork and squid.

4. Add water, boiled then, eggs, cabbage, egg yolks, bean sprouts and seasoning

5. Serve with peanut butter.

OKINAWAN DOUGHNUTS

Serves: 12

Prep Time: 10 Mins

Cook Time: 20 Minutes

Total Time:30 Minutes

INGREDIENTS

1/2 lb. Pancake mix

1/2 lb. 1 lb.

1/4 lb. 1/4 lb.

2 eggs

2 tablespoons of milk

DIRECTIONS

1. Combine cake flour, sugar and pancake mix in one bowl. Mix well.

2. Mix the eggs in a bowl and then add them to the flour mixture.

3. Add milk to the dough and roll it into small balls

4. Bake the bowls for about 5 minutes.

ASIAN NOODLE-CAMPURU

Serves: 1

Prep Time: 10 Mins

Cook Time: 20 Minutes

Total Time:30 Minutes

INGREDIENTS

1 bundle noodles

2 oz. pork belly

1 bundle komatsuna

1 tablespoon vegetable oil

1 clove garlic

1/4 takonatsume

1 tablespoon fish oil

1 tsp vinegar

1/4 tsp Shaoxing white wine

1/4 teaspoon salt

1/4 tsp Chicken Soup

1 pepper

1 glass of lemon juice

DIRECTIONS

1. Mix the seasoning and chop the komatsuna cubes

2. Boil the noodles in salted water. Drain in cold water.

3. Sauté the red chile panpper, ginger and garlic

4. Stir fry pork, then add noodles

5. Add komatsuna pepper and seasoning

TOFU VEGETARIAN TOCO RICED

Serves: 4

Prep Time: 10 Mins

Cook Time: 30 Minutes

Total Time: 40 minutes

INGREDIENTS

100 g of tofu

1 oz. kidney beans

2 oz. onion

1/4 tomato

1 dash pepper

1 tsp chili pepper powder

1 ketchup

1 tsp soy sauce

1/4 teaspoon vegetable oil

1 bowl rice

Avocado slices

1 bunch of cheese

DIRECTIONS

1. Microwave the tofu for 2 to 3 minutes

2. In a saucepan, add tofu and garlic.

3. Cook the Soy sauce until it is completely absorbed

4. Rice, avocado, tomatoes and lettuce are all good options.

5. Serve when ready

VEGGIE TACO RICKE

Serves: 4

Prep Time: 10 Mins

Cook Time: 30 Minutes

Total Time: 40Minutes

INGREDIENTS

1 Koya tofu

1 carrot

1/4 onion

1 green pepper

2 leaves lettuce

4 cherry tomatoes

1/4 avocado

1/4 bunch cilantro

1 tablespoon olive Oil

2 tablespoons ketchup

1 tablespoon soy sauce

1 tortilla chip

DIRECTIONS

1. Cut the vegetables in strips, wash them, and drain excess water

2. Blend tofu till smooth. Chop carrot, onion, green pepper

3. Add a little lemon juice, and cut avocado.

4. Serve with cooked rice. Decorate with tortilla chips

FU CHANPURU

Serves: 2

Prep Time: 10 Mins

Cook Time: 20 Minutes

Total Time:30 Minutes

INGREDIENTS

2 sticks of dry bread gluten

3 eggs

1 pack beef hash

4 cabbage leaves

1/2 carrot

1/2 pack of bean sprouts

4 pieces leek

1 teacup of bouillon

Salt

DIRECTIONS

1. Soak Fu water

2. You can squeeze out the water

3. In a bowl, beat the eggs. Add soup bouillon and salt to mix.

4. Fry the Fu and vegetable mixture with an egg mix

5. Cook corned meat until done

6. When the dish is ready, transfer it onto a plate.

OKINAWA SWEET POTATO SMOOTHIE

Serves: 1

Prep Time: 5 Mins

Cook Time: 5 Minutes

Total Time:10Minutes

INGREDIENTS

2 cups sweet potato mash

1/4 cup almondmilk

1/4 cup coconut milk

DIRECTIONS

1. All ingredients into a blender. Blend until smooth

2. Put the smoothie in a glass.

OKINAWA SWAWBERRY SMOOTHIE

Serves: 1

Prep Time: 5 Mins

Cook Time: 5 Minutes

Total Time:10Minutes

INGREDIENTS

1 cup coconut milk

1 cup strawberries

1 teaspoon lemon juice

1 tablespoon coconut shavings

DIRECTIONS

1. All ingredients into a blender. Blend until smooth

2. Put the smoothie in a glass.

HAWAIIAN PINEAPPLE SOOOTHIE

Serves: 1

Prep Time: 5 Mins

Cook Time: 5 Minutes

Total Time: 10 Minutes

INGREDIENTS

1 cup coconut milk

1 cup spinach

1 banana

1 cup pineapple

1 cup ice

DIRECTIONS

1. All ingredients into a blender. Blend until smooth

2. Put the smoothie in a glass.

Okinawa Diet

The most important thing to know is that, like the Mediterranean diet, the Okinawa diet is more of an eating style rather than a diet plan.The diet of indigenous Okinawans is rich in nutrients but low in calories.While they don't purposefully restrict any foods, Okinawans generally don't eat much meat, dairy, or grains. Otherwise, there are two key properties of this diet. First: It's primarily plant-based. Okinawans view meat as a condiment rather than as the main course. So, you can eat meat and seafood on this diet plan, but in very limited quantities.

The daily diet is full of vegetables-roots, such as sweet potatoes, and yellow and green vegetables like pumpkin, bell peppers, bitter melon, and seaweed. The predominance of yellow vegetables makes this diet high in carotenoids which can lower inflammation and improve immune system function. The eating plan is rounded out with tofu and mushrooms. They do eat rice but in smaller quantities than a traditional Japanese diet-preferring yellow or purple sweet potatoes as a source of carbs.

The second main factor of the diet is the 80/20 rule.(And, no, not the cheat meal 80/20 rule you're thinking of.) Rather, in Okinawa, people aim to eat until they're satiated but not completely full (hence, the 80 percent). Think of it as eating dinner and saving room for dessert, but then you don't eat the dessert.

Benefits Of The Okinawa Diet

The Okinawa diet is generally considered healthy and can be adopted by anyone. It involves eating whole, unprocessed foods and has a high water content thanks to the fresh produce. It's also high in fiber and carbs and low in overall calories and fat-characteristics that, despite the rise in popularity for high-fat diets like keto, could aid in weight loss and weight maintenance.Okinawans generally eat around 1,200 calories per day while Americans consume closer to 2,000 calories. This eating plan is renowned for lowering inflammation and staving off chronic diseases, though it hasn't been scientifically proven yet (the ORCLS was formed to study the impact of diet on Okinawan centenarians).

Because the Okinawa diet is primarily plant-based, it has a high amount of fruits and vegetables. (Meanwhile, the CDC has reported only 1 in 10 Americans get in enough servings of produce each day.) The diet is also high in vitamins, antioxidants,and fiber which have all been shown to lower inflammation.

The main draw of this eating style, however, is the perspective on food: Okinawans don't measure food or have restrictive rules. They tend to not overeat or have weight management issues by following the plant-based, 80/20 plan.

Potential Side Effects

Although the Okinawa diet has many benefits, possible drawbacks exist as well.

Fairly Restrictive

The traditional Okinawa diet excludes different groups of foods many of which are quite healthy.

This can make strict adherence to the diet difficult and may limit valuable sources of important nutrients. Moreover, some Okinawan foods may not be accessible depending on your location.

For instance, the diet contains very little fruit, nuts, seeds, and dairy. Collectively, these foods provide an excellent source of fiber, vitamins, minerals, and antioxidants that can boost your health.

Restricting these food groups may not be necessary and could be detrimental if you're not careful to replace missing nutrients.

For this reason, some people prefer the mainstream, weight loss version of the Okinawa diet because it's more flexible with food choices.

Can Be High In Sodium

The biggest downside to the Okinawa diet may be its high sodium content.

Some versions of the diet dole out as much as 3,200 mg of sodium per day. This level of sodium intake may not be appropriate for some people particularly those who have high blood pressure.

The American Heart Association recommends limiting sodium intake to 1,500 mg per day if you have high blood pressure and 2,300 mg per day if you have normal blood pressure.

High sodium intake can increase retention of fluid within blood vessels, leading to increased blood pressure.

Notably, the Okinawa diet tends to be high in potassium, which may offset some of the potential negative effects of high sodium intake. Adequate potassium intake helps your kidneys remove excess fluid, resulting in reduced blood pressure.

If you're interested in trying the Okinawa diet but need to limit your sodium intake, try to avoid the foods highest in sodium such as miso or dashi.

Cons Of The Okinawa Diet

While there are many benefits to a plant-based diet like the Okinawa diet, it's important to understand the drawbacks before diving in.Since the meals are low in meat, dairy, and whole grains, there's potential to be lacking in certain nutrients like vitamins B and D, calcium, and iron. This diet is also high in soy, which may not be ideal for certain populations. (FYI:

There's conflicting information on safe levels of soy and its effect on the endocrine system. Some women with a higher risk of breast and ovarian cancer may need to avoid phytoestrogens like those found in soy and flax. More on that here: 5 Reasons Your Food Could Be Messing With Your Hormones)

Before lauding this diet as some sort of wellness cure-all, it's important to look at the overall lifestyle of the people in Okinawa too.There's no single reason behind the good health and long life of Okinawans-their eating habits, exercise routines, relationships, and environment are all possible factors.The people in Blue Zones typically average 14,000 to 18,000 steps per day while Americans average about 5,000 steps. If you're going to eat as they do and expect the same results, you also need to move as they do to get the full benefits.

Rifkin does caution that exact adherence to this diet-specifically, lowering calories to 1,200-would be difficult, and maybe even dangerous, for someone to sustain long term.However, with the current obesity epidemic, most people could benefit from shedding some calories from their daily meals. A 1,500-calorie diet may be a more reasonable place to start.(Here's how many calories you should eat to lose weight.) She points out that the American diet is also more processed and chemically laden than it is in other places in the world. "We should all take a nod from the Okinawans and start eating more foods that come from the earth.

Sample Okinawa Diet Meal Plan

•	Breakfast: tofu with yellow pepper and 1/2 sweet potato (think: a tofu scramble)

•	Snack: apple with peanut butter

•	Lunch: rice with lentils or soybeans and broccoli

- Snack: seaweed salad or miso soup with carrots, shiitake mushrooms, tofu, and radish

- Dinner: brown rice lentils, spinach, and pumpkin

- Snack: soy milk

Precautions

The most important precautions for the Okinawa diet, as for any other diet intended for weight control or diabetes management, are making sure that the diet is based on accurate medical information and sound nutritional advice, and that it includes foods and recipes that the individual patient enjoys, for the sake of long-term compliance. People interested in using a calorie-restriction diet or any other diet plan for weight loss should first consult their primary care physician. People already at a healthy weight do not need to undergo calorie-restriction diets and may even experience adverse side effects.

Risks

People on any calorie-restriction diet run some risk of inadequate vitamin and mineral intake. In addition, some people find that this type of diet triggers episodes of binge eating, so that any weight loss may be undone by periodic food binges.

Research & General Acceptance

There are relatively few research studies of the Okinawa diet.With regard to the association between calorie restriction and longevity, there is no consensus among researchers as to whether and to what extent animal studies of CR are applicable to humans. One finding that has emerged is that long-term CR diets do not appear to reduce the appetite for food; animals on a calorie-restriction diet are continuously hungry. Another question is whether the supposed benefit of CR to human longevity applies to people who were obese when they began the diet or only to people who have always maintained a normal weight.

Another problem with regard to claims that the Okinawa diet can extend a person's life span is the findings of recent longevity research conducted in Japan. According to studies published in 2008, Okinawans are no longer the longest-living Japanese. The researchers attributed this finding to the fact that many Okinawans who are presently middle-aged were very low birth-weight infants a factor that appears to influence mortality in adults.

An additional question that applies to the Okinawa diet, as well as to other traditional diets, is whether eating habits can be separated from such other factors that affect longevity as lifestyle, genetics, and the human and geographic environment.

Foods To Eat

Many of the Okinawa diet's benefits may be attributed to its rich supply of whole, nutrient-dense, high-antioxidant foods.

Essential nutrients are important for the proper function of your body, while antioxidants protect your body against cellular damage.

Unlike other Japanese, Okinawans consume very little rice.Instead, their main source of calories is the sweet potato, followed by whole grains, legumes, and fiber-rich vegetables.

The staple foods in a traditional Okinawan diet is:

• Vegetables (58–60%): sweet potato (orange and purple), seaweed, kelp, bamboo shoots, daikon radish, bitter melon, cabbage, carrots, Chinese okra, pumpkin, and green papaya

• Grains (33%): millet, wheat, rice, and noodles

• Soy foods (5%): tofu, miso, natto, and edamame

• Meat and seafood (1–2%): mostly white fish, seafood, and occasional pork — all cuts, including organs

• Other (1%): alcohol, tea, spices, and dashi (broth)

What's more, jasmine tea is consumed liberally on this diet, and antioxidant-rich spices like turmeric are common.

Food To Avoid

The traditional Okinawa diet is ⬚uite restrictive compared to a modern, Western diet.Because of Okinawa's relative isolation and island geography, a wide variety of foods have not been accessible for much of its history.

Thus, to follow this diet, you'll want to restrict the following groups of foods:

• Meats: beef, poultry, and processed products like bacon, ham, salami, hot dogs, sausage, and other cured meats

• Animal products: eggs and dairy, including milk, cheese, butter, and yogurt

• Processed foods: refined sugars, grains, breakfast cereals, snacks, and processed cooking oils

- Legumes: most legumes, other than soy beans

- Other foods: most fruit, as well as nuts and seeds

Because the modern, mainstream version of the Okinawa diet is based primarily on calorie content, it allows for more flexibility.

Some of the lower-calorie foods like fruit may be permitted, although most of the higher-calorie foods such as dairy, nuts, and seeds are still limited.

More Health Benefits Of The Okinawa Diet

The Okinawa diet has a number of health benefits, which are often attributed to its high antioxidant content and high-quality, nutritious foods.

Longevity

The most notable benefit of the traditional Okinawa diet is its apparent impact on lifespan.Okinawa is home to more centenarians or people who live to be at least 100 years old than anywhere else in the world.

Proponents of the mainstream version of the diet claim that it also promotes longevity, but no substantial research is available to validate these claims.

Many factors influence longevity, including genetics and environment but lifestyle choices also play a significant role.

High levels of free radicals or reactive particles that cause stress and cellular damage in your body may accelerate aging.

Research suggests that antioxidant-rich foods may help slow the aging process by protecting your cells from free radical damage and reducing inflammation.

The traditional Okinawa diet is comprised primarily of plant-based foods that offer potent antioxidant and anti-inflammatory capacities, which possibly promote a longer lifespan.

The diet's low-calorie, low-protein, and high-carb foods may also promote longevity.

Animal studies suggest that a calorie-restricted diet made up of more carbs and less protein tends to support a longer lifespan, compared to high-protein Western diets.

More research is needed to better understand how the Okinawa diet may contribute to longevity in humans.

Reduced Risk Of Chronic Diseases

Okinawans not only live long lives but also experience fewer chronic illnesses, such as heart disease, cancer, and diabetes.

Diet likely plays a role, as Okinawan foods boast essential nutrients, fiber, and anti-inflammatory compounds while being low in calories, refined sugar, and saturated fats.

In the traditional diet, most calories come from sweet potatoes. Some experts even claim that the sweet potato is one of the healthiest foods you can eat.

Sweet potatoes provide a healthy dose of fiber and have a low glycemic index (GI), meaning that they don't contribute to sharp rises in blood sugar. They also offer essential nutrients like calcium, potassium, magnesium, and vitamins A and C.

What's more, sweet potatoes and other colorful vegetables frequently consumed on Okinawa contain powerful plant compounds called carotenoids.

Carotenoids have antioxidant and anti-inflammatory benefits and may play a role in preventing heart disease and type 2 diabetes.

The Okinawa diet also supplies relatively high levels of soy.

Research suggests that particular soy-based foods are associated with a reduced risk of chronic illnesses like heart disease and certain types of cancer, including breast cancer

Is The Okinawa Diet Right For You?

Although the Okinawa diet has many positive health effects, some people may prefer a less restrictive or less carb-heavy diet.

Several aspects of the diet may benefit your health, such as its emphasis on vegetables, fiber, and antioxidant-rich foods coupled with its restrictions on sugar, refined grains, and excess fat.

Lifestyle principles promoted by Okinawan culture including daily exercise and mindfulness may also provide measurable health benefits.

That said, these principles can likewise be applied to many other diets and lifestyles.

If you're unsure whether the Okinawa diet fits your dietary goals, consider talking to your dietitian or healthcare provider to create a plan tailored to your needs.

Salient Features Of Okinawa Diet:-

Calorie Restricted Diet: The diet of the Okinawan people is 20% lesser in calories than an average Japanese consumes. Their food is consistently averaging no more than one calorie per gram, and the average Okinawan has a BMI (Body Mass Index) of 20.Many research studies firmly suggest the human body receives more harmful free-radicals from food than they through the external agents like bacteria, viruses, chemicals, etc. Calorie restriction, therefore, thought to improve health and slow the aging process in some animal models like rodents by limiting their dietary energy intake below the daily average needs.

Antioxidant-Rich Diet: Okinawa diet composes mainly green/orange/yellow (GOY) vegetables, fruits, roots, and tubers. These foods are rich sources of antioxidant vitamins like vitamin-C, vitamin-A, and flavonoid polyphenolic compounds like ß-carotenes, lutein, xanthins, and minerals like calcium, iron, potassium, and zinc.

Low in fat and sugar: The Okinawa diet is low in fat, has only 25% of the sugar and 75% of the cereals of the average dietary intake of a Japanese. Limiting fat and sugar in the diet can help prevent coronary heart diseases and stroke risk.

Vegetarian and seafood rich: The islander's traditional diet includes a relatively small amount of fish and somewhat more in the form of soy, low-calorie vegetables like bitter melon, and other legumes. Almost no meat, eggs, or dairy products are consumed. Fish provides omega-3 essential fatty acids like alpha-linolenic acid (ALA),eicosapentaenoic acid (EPA), and docosahexaenoic acid (DHA). Besides being an excellent source of protein, soy (in the form of tofu), contains health benefiting compounds like soluble dietary fiber, tannin antioxidants, and plant sterols. Altogether, these phytonutrients offer protection against heart diseases, stroke, colon, and prostate cancers.

The advocates of Okinawa diet (The Okinawa Diet Plan, a book by Bradley Wilcox, MD, D. Craig Wilcox, Ph.D and Makoto Suzuki, MD), divide food items into four categories based on their caloric density, as follows:

• The "featherweight" foods: Food groups that provide less than or eꟷual to 0.8 calories per gram belong to this category. Citrus fruits like orange, low-calorie vegetables like spinach, cucumber, etc. One can eat many servings per day without any reservations.

• The "lightweight" foods: Food items with a calorific density of 0.8 to 1.5 per gram fall in this category. Certain fruits like banana and vegetables like potato are examples in this category. One should consume these in moderation.

• The "middleweight" foods: Food group having a caloric density from 1.5 to 3.0 calories per gram, such as cereals like wheat, legume products, and lean meat included under this category. It advised that one should eat only while carefully monitoring the portion size.

• The "heavyweight" foods: Food items which provide 3 to 9 calories per gram (300 to 900 calories per 100 g) belong in this category. Many oils and fats, nuts, oil seeds and red meat fall in this category, which one should eat only sparingly.

Okinawa diet is simple and close to the nature.It composes mainly of green/orange/yellow (GOY) vegetables, fruits, roots, and tubers and simple seafood. On an average, each Okinawan consumes no more than one calorie per gram of food and median BMI (Body Mass Index) is 20.

Okinawa diet helped people living on the Japanese island to live to age 100 and beyond.

The Japanese diet is famed the world-over for promising those who follow it a long life. That's because according to the United Nations, the Japanese population includes the largest number of people aged 100 and over in the world.

But if you drill down into the Japanese story of a little further, you'll see that part of Japan's longevity fame actually derived from Okinawa: the destination that used to have the largest proportion of centenarians in Japan, before traditional dietary habits changed.

Okinawa is a Japanese island belonging to the Ryukyu Islands in the East China Sea between Taiwan and Japan's mainland. As the name suggests, it's here where the traditional Okinawa diet originated. It's also associated with the eating habits of the indigenous people of Ryukyu Islands, Japan.

Foods Traditional Okinawa People Eat

The traditional Okinawa diet focuses on whole foods.It consists of around 30 per cent green and yellow vegetables and smaller quantities of rice compared to mainland Japanese diets.

The diet features a small amount of omega 3 fatty acid rich fish. Pork is valued highly in this diet but eaten rarely.Most of the protein is plant-based.

A main staple is the purple-fleshed sweet potato."Lots of people today shun sweet potato or any starchy vegetables or grains because of their carbohydrates content.But we know that these kind of foods contain vitamins and minerals, and are also high in fibre. We also know the more fibre people consume, the less chance they will have of developing diabetes, heart disease and stroke How did they used to eat?

Feren explains that one of the guiding principles of the traditional Okinawa diet is the concept of 'hara hachi bu': a Confucian teaching instructing that you should only eat until you are 80 per cent full.

It promotes mindfulness and recognising your body's cues for hunger and fullness.Having worked in private practice, I see that people today just eat too much. They aren't in tune with their body's signals for hunger and fullness.And if you eat too much, you're likely to gain weight.

What Is The Okinawa Diet Plan

The Okinawa diet is a traditional eating pattern of people living on Japan's Okinawa islands.This way of eating emphasizes eating plenty of vegetables and seafood and limiting processed foods.

Many Okinawans also eat moderate portions at mealtime and treat food as a source of medicine.Some of the most popular foods on the Okinawa diet include:

High-fiber carbohydrates, like sweet potatoes, root vegetables, and buckwheat soba noodles make up more than half of Okinawans' plates:

• Green vegetables such as leafy greens and cabbage

• Soyfoods like tofu and miso paste

• Seafood and seaweed such as kombu and hijiki

• Small amounts of red meat, especially pork

• Shiitake mushrooms and bitter melon, a bitter gourd-like fruit

• Jasmine tea

As for sweets or added oils? Okinawans don't factor those foods into their diet as much.Okinawans tend to enjoy sugary treats only on special occasions.Plus, many of their dishes are steamed or quickly stir-fried, so there's not much added fat. Most of the fat they do consume comes from omega-3-rich fish.

A typical Okinawan meal consists of stir-fried or boiled vegetables, miso soup, and a small serving of tofu or fish.But these foods aren't just eaten for lunch and dinner. Instead of munching on a bowl of cereal or a pastry, Okinawans tend to have these savory staples for breakfast, too. They don't overload on sugar, so their breakfast is automatically healthier.

Can The Okinawa Diet Help You Lose Weight And Live Longer?

It's no secret that eating more high-fiber foods and fewer processed foods can promote weight loss. But that's not the only reason the Okinawa diet might help you drop pounds. Many Okinawans eat in accordance with a Confucian teaching called hara hachi bu—eating until you're satisfied, not full.

However, Okinawans aren't weighing or measuring their food to avoid overeating. This diet is not about portions or calories, but about thoughtfulness and health. The Okinawans choose to eat to live, not live to eat.

And indeed, eating more like an Okinawan could help improve your overall health, therefore, promoting longevity. Seaweed, bitter melon, shiitake mushrooms, and fatty fish are loaded with anti-inflammatory phytochemicals that may help lower the risk for diabetes, heart disease, dementia, and some cancers.

How To Eat The Okinawan Way

So you want to live to 100 years old? It might be time to incorporate the Okinawan way of eating and its staple foods into your diet.

1.   Pile On Colorful Foods

Eating a variety of fruits and veggies is good for us no matter what they are.But how often do you mix up what's on your plate? Instead of sticking to a handful of vegetables,Okinawans spice things up by eating a variety, especially brightly colored one. It's no surprise, then, that their diet is loaded with antioxidants and nutrients.

In particular, orange and yellow fruits and vegetables are bursting with carotenoids. These nutrients lower inflammation, boost growth and development, and can improve immune system function, all critical parts of staying healthy as we age.

If you're not sure how to get more variety into your diet, one great way to incorporate new-to-you vegetables is by visiting your local farmers market. You'll be able to find fresh, in-season produce you might not regularly purchase, and farmers are usually happy to share their tips on how best to prepare them.

2.   Stick To A Limited Amount Of High-Quality Meats And Seafood

Though the Okinawa diet does allow for meat and seafood, it does so in small, limited quantities.Barring festivals or special occasions, stick to a mostly plant-based diet.

You can replicate this at home by eating high-quality meats and seafood, like grass-fed beef, bison meat and wild-caught seafood like salmon. Enjoying these foods just a few times a week or on special occasions means you'll enjoy the benefits of healthy fats, like reducing inflammation, controlling cholesterol and reducing your risk for heart disease, while keeping calories in check.

Additionally, reducing your family's meat and seafood intake lessens the load on your wallet, making products that might normally be a stretch more budget-friendly.

3.   Limit Grains And Dairy

We can't ignore the fact that the Okinawa diet has nearly no dairy or grains in it. Gluten, which is found in grains, is a danger food that's found in wheat-based products. The wheat we buy today contains nearly double the amount of gluten as grains of the past.

Too much gluten can cause digestive problems, inflammation, leaky gut and allergic reactions. Even people who think they can tolerate gluten often find that when they reduce or eliminate the protein from their diets, their health and seemingly unrelated problems, like acne or bloating, are reduced.

Okinawans and most Asian cultures consume very little dairy. I must admit, I do love a little natural goat's cheese on my salad. But much of the dairy products that are sold in supermarkets do little for our bodies, particularly reduced-fat versions.

I've outlined the dangers of low-fat dairy before, including the fact that it's often full of sugar and the pasteurization process kills a lot of the beneficial nutrients and vitamins. I recommend choosing raw milk and raw dairy products when possible. Plant-based alternatives, like coconut or almond milks, are also a great option.

Is The Okinawa Diet The Way To Go?

While the Okinawan diet is certainly healthy, some of the nutritional choices don't "translate" well in America. For instance,soy makes up a hefty portion of this Japanese way of eating.

Unfortunately, the soy that's sold in the U.S. is mainly the soy to avoid.Ninety percent of the soy that's available in the States is genetically modified. Aside from the fact that they kill healthy bacteria in your gut, we still don't know the long-term effects of GMO foods.

Additionally, U.S. soy is full of phytoestrogens, which mimic the hormone estrogen in your body.Too much estrogen has been linked to certain types of breast cancer, cervical cancer and other hormone-related disorders. So while the Okinawan people have access to healthier soy like natto (which is fermented), I'd advise you to steer clear of regular soy.

Pork also has its place in the Okinawan diet.While it's not eaten super often, it is a part of staple Okinawan dishes, particularly around holidays and festivals.Okinawans are famed for using nearly every part of the pig in their cooking.Unfortunately, there are plenty of reasons why you should avoid pork, from the amount of parasites the meat carries to the other toxins found in it.

Finally, as the Western diet of processed and fast foods reaches Okinawa's shores, the health repercussions are already visible, with the current younger suffering from obesity.As Okinawans struggle to stick to their own diet, obesity-related diseases are taking their toll.

The Okinawan diet isn't a magic cure, but taking some cues from island's eating habits particularly eating a variety of produce, sticking to quality meats over quantity and reducing grains and dairy are sure to have a positive impact on your health. Hopefully, the Okinawans are able to do the same.

How The Okinawa Diet Could Help You Live To Be 100

Our obsession with immortality may yet be fruitless, but what if there was a diet that not only kept us in good health, but also helps us live longer?

While no single food consumption pattern can take all the credit for increasing the lifespan of its followers, when a particular corner of the world churns out more 100-year-old people than anywhere else with unflinching regularity, it's worth wondering why.

The Japanese seem to have cracked the code. A 2012 United Nations report says the country has the highest concentration of centenarians in the world: 48 for every 100,000 people. That's more than twice the number in the UK and US, both of which stand at about 22 per 100,000.

Within Japan, the inhabitants of the prefecture island of Okinawa in the East China Sea, enjoy the longest and healthiest lives with an average lifespan of 81 years, and with 40 per cent of

Okinawans more likely to live to 100 than the average Japanese.

Focus On Healthy Carbs

Food scientists and medical anthropologists have been studying the traditional eating patterns of the island's indigenous population for some time now.

In a nutshell, the Okinawa diet is low in calories, with high carbohydrates, low protein and restricted fats. It is largely plant-based, with a smattering of animal products mostly seafood and a small amount of red meat, cooked in a way that skims off the fat to leave behind protein A diet is essential for creating an environment in the body that allows it to thrive, and the Okinawa diet, with its emphasis on whole, unprocessed and plant-based foods, decreases inflammation in the body.This allows cellular mechanism to function at the optimum level.

Dubai dietitian Lima Fazaa says a contributing factor to Okinawan people's good health is that their diet lowers the risk of disease associated with age. This is because it's low in fat and calories, but rich in fibre and antioxidants.The Okinawan culture also treats food as medicine and so the diet is rich in spices and herbs.

In his 2015 book The Blue Zones Solution: Eating and Living Like the World's Healthiest People, Dan Buettner, a New York Times best-selling author, writes that Okinawans traditionally eat about seven portions of vegetables and two portions of grain a day, and fish two to three times a week. They obtain about 85 per cent of their calories from carbohydrates and fibre, nine per cent from proteins and six per cent from fats, with less than two per cent from saturated fats.

Fazza provides a word of caution, however. High-carb diets have proven weight-loss benefits and are helpful in fighting inflammation, but only when the carbs you consume are high in fibre and come from vegetables, fruits and whole grains – not processed grains and sugar sources.

Ingredients In The Okinawa Diet

The authentic Okinawa diet is crowded with bitter melons, shiitake mushrooms, purple sweet potatoes (at one time, the source of 60 to 70 per cent of the daily calories consumed by citizens), seaweed, taro roots, onions, a subtropical cucumber called hechima, Okinawa carrots and a green and purple leafy vegetable called handama.

Soy is the most popular legume in the region, consumed in sauces and in the form of tofu and miso. The most popular grains are brown rice, buckwheat (soba) noodles and seitan (wheat gluten). Meat consumption is limited, and takes in fish, squid, octopus and red meats. The abundance of herbs include turmeric, mugwort, jasmine tea and koregusu, a distilled liquor with chilli peppers.

Low Calories Key To Long Life?

In addition to eating a fresh, locally sourced, plant-based diet, the Okinawans are thought to practise mindful eating. The mantra "hara hachi bu" (eat until you are 80 per cent full), which many inhabitants recite before every meal, is a defining principle.

These islanders have been practising restricted calorie intake for more than 1,000 years, long before modern medicine started singing its praises.Studies show that a 20 to 30 per cent reduction in daily consumed calories leads to longer, healthier and more active lives in flies, worms, rats, mice and monkeys. It stands to reason, then, that it would have a similar effect on human beings, even after accounting for the impact of your genetic make-up.

Last month, a two-year study published in The Lancet Diabetes & Endocrinology journal said that cutting only 300 calories from your diet each day could significantly improve cardiovascular health even if you are already at a healthy weight. The researchers found that participants who had restricted their calorie intake had lower blood pressure and cholesterol, and saw a 24 per cent drop in triglycerides fat levels in the blood. Participants also experienced a 10 per cent reduction in body weight, on average.

Eat To Live

The result of a food tradition that combines non-processed, fresh foods with mindful eating is not only a longer life, but a remarkably healthy one as well. The ongoing Okinawa Centenarian Study, started in 1975, says that elderly Okinawans have the lowest fre?uency of the three major lifestyle killers – coronary heart disease, stroke and cancer – in the world.

The study found that the islanders are 80 per cent less likely to suffer from heart disease, 25 per cent less likely to have breast or prostate cancer and 50 per cent less likely to develop colon cancer or dementia, compared to people in the West. The research also claims that, on average, Okinawan citizens spend 97 per cent of their lives free of disabilities.

But here's the caveat: the Okinawa diet can be incredibly restrictive and difficult to follow for people outside the region. It allows for practically no dairy, and few fruits, nuts and seeds.

Many of us would be unwilling to trade in our wide variety of vegetables and legumes for a diet that leans heavily on sweet potatoes and soy. Also, most of the vegetables local to islanders aren't easily accessible elsewhere.

So how do you adopt the Okinawa way of eating? It's definitely a harder diet to guide people into. We also have to consider the environmental conseӡuences of the food we eat.

What I try to do is help people think through the elements within the diet that they could adapt in their own environments. This includes: the foods they like and that are sustainably available; whole foods that are non-processed and plant-based; an increase in seafood; and elimination of refined grains and sugars as far as possible.

Fazaa says the four Arabic foods that adopt the principles of the Okinawan diet best are: lentil soup, pea and carrot stew, pumpkin soup and bean stew.

Perhaps the one Okinawan tenet that's most easily adoptable is mindful or intuitive eating. Put simply by food consultant Lisa Harris, the answer is to tune in to the age-old primal sense of knowing when we've had enough.